"After over twenty years of yo-yo dieting and feeling hopeless to ever get a grip on my weight, I am so happy to have found Monica's book. I followed her method of changing my thinking about food and my body for a few months now, and can hardly believe how easily the weight has come off! I've lost a total of twenty pounds and am currently at my ideal weight! My husband sees that I am not dieting, and keeps asking me, 'What is your secret?' I have to laugh, realizing that I am actually living the "secret" of my naturally skinny friends! This book has been life-changing and I am forever grateful."

—Judy, Honolulu

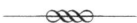

"As both a college student facing the pressures of expectations, and as a teenage girl who has played (and lost) the game of comparison over and over, I can honestly say this book is freeing. An exposé from someone who has been there and who understands, *The Secret to My Naturally Skinny Friends* speaks truth about a difficult and misunderstood topic and brings life to a place of despair and inadequacy."

—Natalie, Texas

The Secret of Your NATURALLY SKINNY FRIENDS

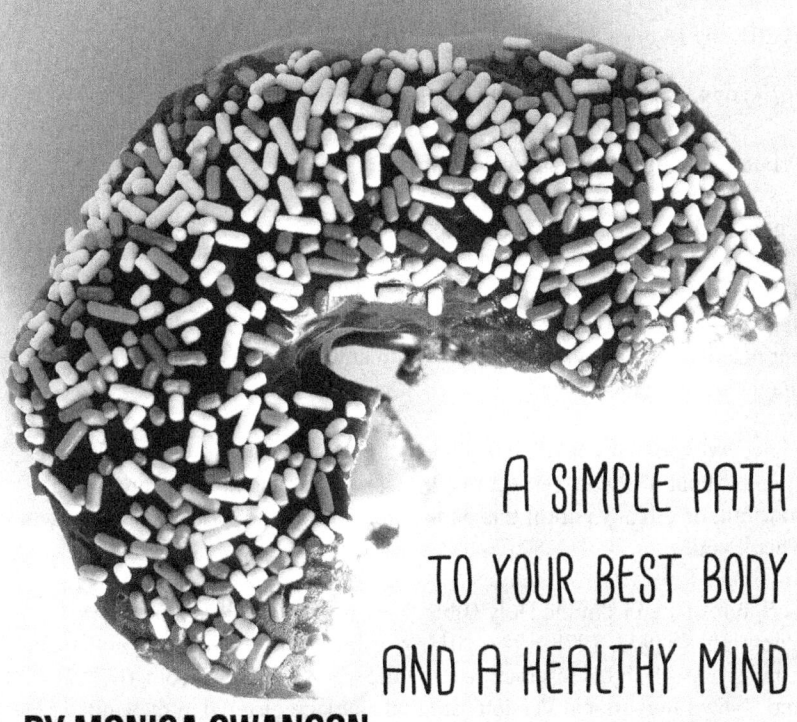

A SIMPLE PATH TO YOUR BEST BODY AND A HEALTHY MIND

BY MONICA SWANSON

© 2015 by Monica Swanson

ISBN 978-1517758103

Printed in the United States of America

Cover Photo, Author Photo, & Graphics: Josiah Swanson

This book is not intended as a substitute for the medical advice of physicians. The reader should regularly consult a physician in matters relating to his/her health and particularly with respect to any symptoms that may require diagnosis or medical attention.

I have worked really hard on this book, and would love for you to tell your friends about it! Please respect my work however, and do not reproduce, transmit, or sell any part of this publication without my prior written consent. Thank you!

Scriptures taken from the Holy Bible, New International Version®, NIV®. Copyright © 1973, 1978, 1984, 2011 by Biblica, Inc.™ Used by permission of Zondervan. All rights reserved worldwide. www.zondervan.com The "NIV" and "New International Version" are trademarks registered in the United States Patent and Trademark Office by Biblica, Inc.™

Table of Contents

- About the Author..6
- Introduction..7
- Ch 1: The Thin Cycle..11
- Ch 2: What's Your Cycle?................................15
- Ch 3: Diets Are Not the Answer......................19
- Ch 4: Four Steps to Real Change 21
    Believe
    Think
    Behave
    Experience

- Ch 5: Practical Tips and Tricks 34
    Challenge: Weight Loss
    Challenge: Exercise Addiction

- Ch 6: The Resistance 39
- Ch 7: Special Occasions, Vacations, and Real Life...42
- Ch 8: Obesity, Special Diets, and General Health.....44
- Ch 9: Five Days in my Life..............................45
- Author's Note...50
- Appendix: The 30-Day Thought Diet 52

monicaswanson.com

ABOUT THE AUTHOR: MONICA SWANSON

Monica lives on the North Shore of Oahu, Hawaii, where she and her husband Dave are raising (and homeschooling) four surfer boys, and a whole bunch of tropical fruit. Monica's background is in Sports Medicine, and she is passionate about family, health, and discovering treasures in every day life. You can find Monica sharing stories, recipes, faith, and inspiration at www.monicaswanson.com

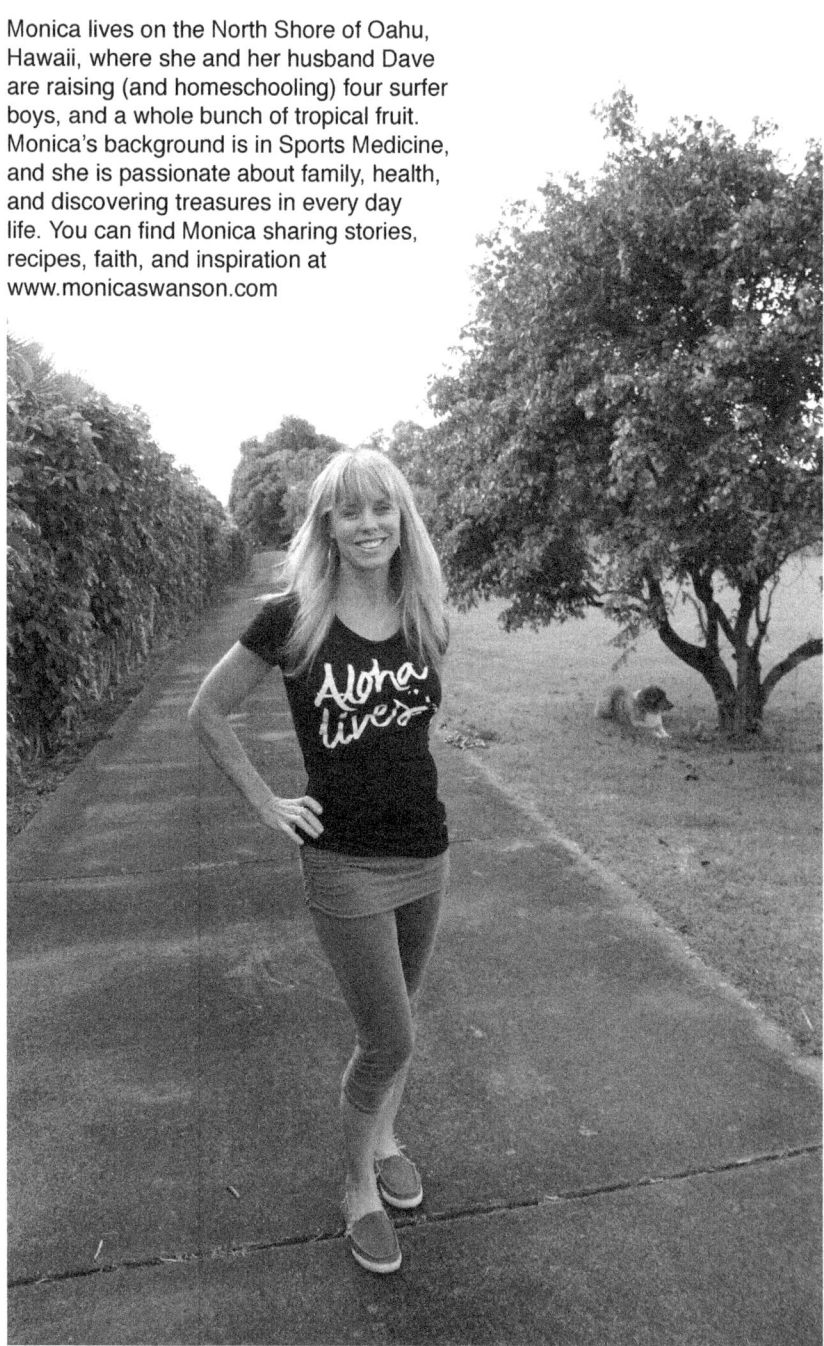

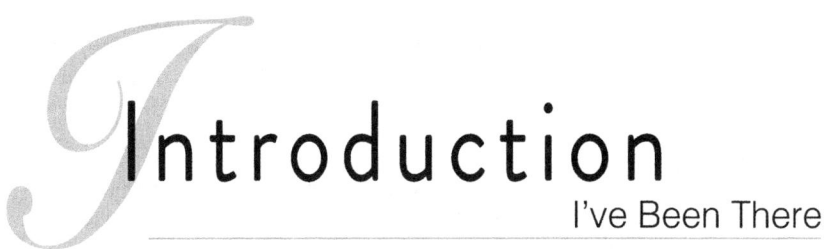

Introduction
I've Been There

If you lie in bed at night recounting everything you ate that day...
If you wake up and rehearse what you might eat the upcoming day...
Or, if you've ever said the words, "I'm going to start my diet on Monday"...
I get you.

If missing a workout makes your world feel out of control...
Or you find yourself comparing your body to everyone you meet...
I feel your pain.

If your moods are affected by your weight...
Or you avoid social settings because you're on a diet or don't want to face the temptation to eat the wrong foods...
I've been there.

If you have have tried diets...
Or taken fat burners...
Or read books hoping to find help but instead find yourself more messed up than before...
I absolutely relate.

But I have good news for you.
I used to do all of that too.
And now I don't.

> **I quit obsessing over food and my body, and ended up weighing less and feeling better than I had before.**

And I believe you can too.

I am writing this book to fulfill a sort of silent vow I made nearly fourteen years ago, when everything changed...

I was 31 years old, and I had spent about half of my life struggling with my relationship with food, exercise and my body. Though I had tried countless diets and exercise programs, nothing solved my problems. I felt like a prisoner in my own mind and body.

My college degree was in Sports Medicine, and I had spent all of my adult life teaching fitness classes and working as a personal trainer. I wished that something in all of that education might provide me with what I needed to establish a healthy relationship with my own body.

But no.

No program I had ever been on – even when they helped me lose body fat or temporarily feel good about myself physically – ever gave me the peace that I longed for. As soon as I lost weight, or met a goal, I became anxious that I might gain it back, or face some situation where I wasn't able to keep up my program.

For seasons, I tried to just embrace myself and love my body however it was, but the truth is that without the tools to change my deepest, habitual thoughts, I would inevitably return to an obsessive focus on myself and my body. **And, frankly, I knew that I felt best and was happiest when I was lean and fit.** Maybe this isn't true for everyone, but I think for most of us it is.

I was envious of friends who seemed to be free in their eating, and never worried about their body. I called them my "naturally skinny" friends, and I wished I was one of them. Instead, I believed that only through stressing and starving and being a slave to my workouts could I keep my weight under control.

Perhaps the most challenging time of all in dealing with these inner battles was during my first two pregnancies. Any moments of control I might have experienced before pregnancy flew out the window as I spent each pregnancy struggling to accept myself and sadly preoccupied with my diet and body. It took away from what should have been a blessed time.

Eventually, I became desperate. I didn't want to continue living as a prisoner any more. It was affecting my marriage and my parenting, and I just hated the daily struggle that had become my normal. So one day I bravely chose to get to the root of the problem, and face the source of my obsessions: my mind.

Because in my most honest place I knew that I wouldn't be free until I figured out how to think differently. After all, no external change had brought me internal peace. I had avoided this all along because simply following another diet or making external changes was much less painful than facing thoughts that were so ingrained in me.

One day I dared to ask myself: "What if those people who I called 'naturally skinny' are really no different than me? Could I be one of them? Could that be possible?" The thought was wild and silly, but even as I asked it a tiny spark of hope sprung up within me.

I set out to tackle my thinking. Being honest about my thought life, and making radical changes to reprogram my thinking was at first very uncomfortable. Downright painful. You'll hear more about the process in future chapters, but the really amazing thing was: as soon as I began the process, I simply knew that I was on the only real road to victory. My confidence grew.

Without anyone to walk with me through this (there was no e-book :)) I had to figure it out as I went. With God's grace, day after day, I began to find a new way to think and to live.

And it was working.

As the weeks passed, I found more and more mental freedom. But something else was happening as well: my body was changing. No, I wasn't gaining weight and losing all sense of control like I had feared. Instead, I felt lighter and healthier. When I finally weighed myself, I was at my ideal weight.

It seemed too good to be true.

> **I wondered: "Why have I spent half of my life obsessing over diets, exercising compulsively, and completely preoccupied with my body, if I actually could achieve my goal weight by letting go of all of that?"**

I felt like I had just discovered a miracle weight loss pill, that was not a pill at all but instead a new way to think! I wanted to tell everyone!

And that is exactly when I promised God and myself that if this was actually for real – if this change that I was making would bring me lasting peace and contentment, (and my ideal body weight to boot!) – then I would be willing to share it with the world.

I just needed to see if it would withstand the test of time.

So I kept practicing the new ways to think. There were some challenging days, but I never turned back. It got easier and easier. I had two more pregnancies over the next 10 years that were a world of difference from the first two. I actually enjoyed the pregnancies, and I gained less weight than I had in the first two, even though I was in my mid- and upper-30s. I celebrated my body, and had no anxiety over my weight.

It has been nearly 14 years since this began. Today I continue to live with complete freedom. In fact, the struggles that filled my mind for 15 years are a distant memory now.

My weight has remained the same.

Best of all, my mind is free, and available for the more important things and people in my life.

So here I am, to follow through on my promise. I want to help anyone that struggles in this area. I am here to give you what I did not have – a hand to hold when you are ready to tackle your issues at the core. I want to tell you that things can get better. You don't have to be a slave to diets or exercise.

You can love and enjoy food… without being *in love* with food.
You can love and enjoy your body… without obsessing over it.

And in the midst of it all, you can achieve your ideal body weight.
In fact, I think the real secret is: your "naturally skinny" friends aren't so different from you after all.

It's time to reclaim your territory.

You can overcome your struggles, and I will show you how!

Take this little quiz to help you decide if this book would be helpful you. Answer Yes or No to the following ten questions:

1. When I wake up, food, diet or something related to that is the first thing on my mind.
2. I often count calories (or carbs, or points, etc.) in the foods that I eat.
3. I have feelings of guilt related to enjoying food.
4. How I feel about my weight affects my moods.
5. When I go to bed at night, I often review what I have eaten during the day.
6. I HAVE to workout to maintain my weight.
7. I feel guilty when I do not exercise for a few days.
8. I have anxiety about not having the ability to exercise (travel, a busy week, etc.)
9. I avoid social settings because of my diet, or how I might be tempted to eat.
10. When I am on vacation or celebrating a special occasion, my eating is different from how it is on an ordinary day.

If you scored YES on even one of the items on this quiz,
I think you'll find useful information in this book!

IMPORTANT NOTE ON JOURNALING:
Before you dive in to read the rest of the book, grab a pen and paper! I have designed each chapter to end with a journaling prompt which will really help and guide you in engaging with this material. I think you will find it a valuable part of this experience!

The Thin Cycle
An Introduction to "The Thin Cycle"

We all have them. Those friends that seem to eat anything they want, and never gain weight. The ones who have never been on a diet, and don't know a calorie from a bump in the road.

Yeah, those. The ones we love to hate.

We tell ourselves that they are "naturally skinny", that they have "good genes". We think there is some secret to why they get to have so much freedom when it comes to food, and we…don't.

But let me ask you a question:
Have you ever actually spent a full day with a "naturally skinny" person?…Have you made careful observations about when/what/how much they are eating?

I have.
And you know what I've found: these "naturally skinny" folks do have a secret.
But it's not what most people think.
It's not their metabolism. (Yes, genetics do play a role – but it's not everything.)
It's not what they eat. "Naturally skinny" people sometimes eat pretty unhealthy foods.
It's not their workouts. Many of them don't exercise at all!

The secret, my friends, is in their *heads*. It's the way they think.

This is how it goes:
"Naturally skinny" people are not *thinking* about food all the time. They are not obsessing over what they *just ate*, what they are *about to eat*, or what *you are eating*.
They really don't care.
"Naturally skinny" people might like food a lot, but they are not *in love* with food.

"Naturally skinny" people have other things on their mind.
They do not have a preoccupation with food. In fact, if you do spend time with these friends, you'll notice that they often forget to eat.

Shocking, I know.

Note: Lest we confuse "naturally skinny" with "problem-free", please keep in mind: these skinny people may have any variety of real-life struggles of their own. *Their issues just don't happen to fall in the food category.*

Food doesn't rule them. Food isn't an issue for them. And therefore, it doesn't have the same pull on them as it might have on someone who is very much focused on their weight, their diet, and *food*.

The result is that "naturally skinny" people actually eat less than the rest of us.

> A note on genetics and metabolism: Our size and shape is absolutely affected by our genetics and our individual metabolism. However, except in certain medical conditions, we all have the ability to alter our body composition through eating less and exercising. Some bodies simply require less food than others. Keep in mind that "skinny," and "thin," are relative terms. (I'll be using "thin" for most of this book because I think it sounds healthier.) One person at their personal healthy and "thin" weight will not look the same as another. This book does not suggest that we all look like supermodels, but that everyone can achieve their own healthy, "thin" place if they chose to.

So – whether they are big-boned or small, short or tall – a person who maintains a lean, healthy weight, and does so without dieting or obsessing, is most likely on what I call the "thin cycle".

These people have a core belief that they are thin...So they think of themselves as thin....(They are not thinking about losing weight)...So they are not obsessed with food...So they eat like a thin person...So they feel *good*...and around and around it goes.

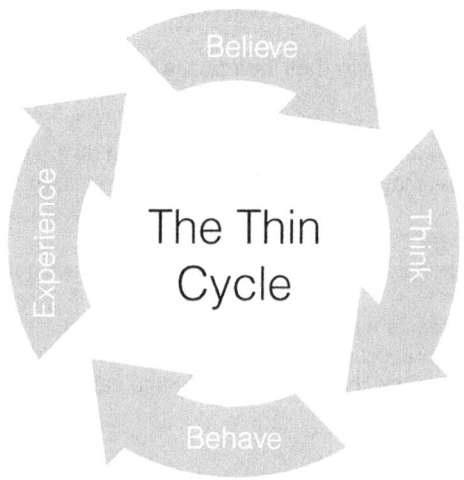

monicaswanson.com

To make even more clear the idea of the **THIN CYCLE**, I will share the story of my friend Christie. Getting to know Christie was actually how I discovered that my own assumption about naturally thin people was totally wrong.

Meet Christie: Christie was a college student in Hawaii who began babysitting for us when my first two boys were young. She was a beautiful girl, with a perfect body as far as I was concerned. Because up to that point I had worked like crazy to try to keep lean and fit, I assumed right away that Christie was into fitness.

But as I got to know her a little bit, it became clear to me that Christie really didn't work out at all.

Next, I concluded that Christie must be a very careful eater – she must follow a strict diet.

Then one day as I was leaving in the morning for an appointment, and I had to switch my car seat to Christie's car, I noticed two very interesting items in her back seat: A skimpy bikini, and....an empty bag of Dunkin' Donuts!

I was so confused. Surely there was a mistake.

But you can be sure that the next time she came over, I went out of my way to peek in her car again.

And the next time, it was different: It was a bikini...and a McDonalds' bag. Unbeknown to the innocent babysitter, I continued to stalk the back of her car, until one day I had to accept the fact that this gorgeous 20-something babysitter...had a terrible diet.

She didn't work out, and she ate donuts and cheeseburgers. *Where was the justice?*

As time went by, I began to observe Christie in more situations...When she would spend time with our family, I would spy on her and notice that though she ate *anything* she felt like, she actually never ate very much. And what's more – she didn't appear to think about the food around her much. She was busy talking, laughing, and chasing kids. She was (to my utter surprise) enjoying life without any true regard to food. Or her body.

Christie chose a coke over a diet coke. She chose a hot dog over fish.

Later, Christie graduated college, got married and moved off the island. By then we were good friends, so we stayed in touch. Over the next years I had begun growing in my own freedom related to diet and my body.

So when I received a phone call about seven years after I had first met Christie, I really wasn't that surprised. Someone had shared a book with her that opened her eyes to all kinds of scientific studies about animal products and your health, and Christie was convinced, and convicted.

Overnight, Christie had become vegan.

With this new found information, Christie was eager to learn more. She continued to read and study health and nutrition and eventually began working for a nutrition company.

So, here is the point of the story: Christie, the Dunkin' Donuts-eating, Coke-drinking, McDonalds-frequenter, had no trouble becoming a vegan because she had never really *loved* food to begin with. She had eaten the way she had because it was easy. And sure – it tasted good. But she wasn't *in love* with any of it. She wasn't obsessive about her food or her body.

Therefore when the information came in, and she felt a personal conviction about what she put in her body, she was able to do a 180 degree turn around without a second thought.

It's been over seven years since that day, and Christie continues to eat very healthy. She works full time for a nutrition company, and teaches yoga. True Story.

Whenever I see Christie I witness that her body looks as amazing as ever. And now she will tell you that she also feels great. She has more energy, and feels really good about the fact that she is taking care of the body that she has always rocked so naturally.

Journal it:

1. Do you know any "naturally skinny" people? Who are they, and what do you know about them? Have you ever observed them for a day? If so, note what you saw about how they ate, exercised, and what was on their mind.

2. Does the Thin Cycle make sense to you? Do you understand how the cycle works and do you see where your "naturally thin" friends might be on it—even if they aren't aware of it?

monicaswanson.com

What's Your Cycle?

Maybe the Thin Cycle does not seem to describe your life.

Perhaps you have spent much of your life on a cycle fueled by negative beliefs and thought patterns.

Wherever you find yourself...negative cycles all begin with a "limiting" belief: these are negative beliefs that you have at some point embraced, which over time have come to define you.

You started **believing** something about yourself...that led to certain **thoughts** about yourself, that led to **behaviors** in your life...that led to how you look, feel, and act like today.

And that my friend, is the premise to this whole book. *(You might go back and re-read that statement.)* **And there's a bonus:** *The same rule applies too every single area of your life.* Don't hesitate to apply it all over the place!

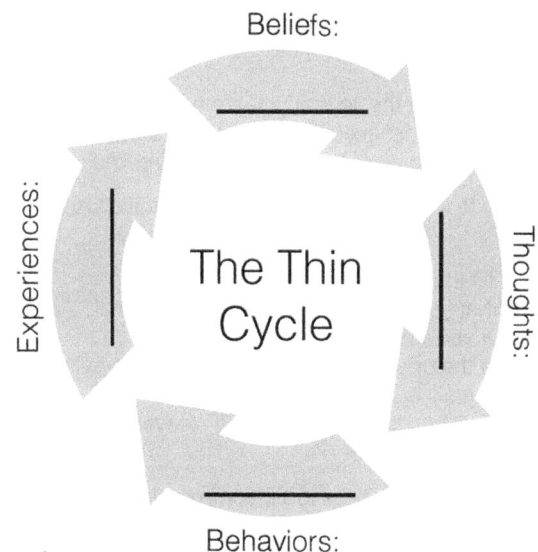

monicaswanson.com

So how does this work itself out?

I'll start with a classic example: if your deep-seated belief is that you are fat, then in the midst of dieting and exercising, you will be faking it at best. At some point, sooner or later, you will experience a gravitational pull back to what you believe in your heart is the "real" you: fat.

No matter the work or discipline, your core beliefs will ultimately rule.

One cheat on the diet and your subconscious begins to shout at you, "See, that's just who you are." One day that the scale doesn't move, (or worse yet, moves in the wrong direction,) and you hear the taunting voice, "See, you'll always be fat."

You go on vacation, and your tendency will be to "take a break" from your diet, because this is "you time," and "you" are not who you are on the diet.

Or on the flip side, you might be doing well on your diet. You might see the scale moving in the right direction. Then what? You experience joy, but joy mixed with fear, knowing this is just temporary. How long could it last? If you're honest, you don't really believe that this thinner you is the "real" you. No, it's more like a fun little body double that just jumped in to congratulate you on all of the hard work of this diet. The "real" you will be back soon, and you just dread her return.

This explains yo-yo dieting. This explains why most people, even doing well on their diet, will gain weight over the holiday season.

> **You will ultimately drift back to who you believe you are.**
> **So the question is:**
> **Who do you really believe you are?**

A negative cycle can come in many forms. There are all kinds of false beliefs that can ensnare a person.

Some of you have accepted the lie that you are not capable of overcoming an *eating disorder*. You have believed that no matter how much you are moving in the right direction, an eating disorder will always define you.

I hope you are ready to identify the false beliefs that have too much influence over your life.

Have you bought a lie that the real you is "fat"?
Have you believed that you will always be "the chubby one".
That you're weak. Or you'll never be athletic?
That you'll always be the one with a sweet tooth, or salt cravings…
Or a carb-addict? It's just "who you are"?
Have you accepted that you'll never wear short sleeves, or a bathing suit?
That those things are for *other people*?

Some people reading this have believed that their value is dependent on the number on a scale. That their self worth comes from fitting someone's expectations of them.

Have you agreed with the negative lables that have defined you?

I hope you feel my blood boil on your behalf, because friends: This is NOT how it's meant to be! You have been lied to and bullied. And you deserve so much more!

Where it all started:

This might be the first time you have been honest with yourself about your deep- seated beliefs, or maybe you've known it all along. It might be uncomfortable to think about.

Rest assured, in Chapter Four we will talk about how to change your core beliefs. But before we get to that, it is important to take an honest look at where your current belief system came from. It will be a lot easier to change your beliefs if you have done the work of honestly looking at the root issues.

The negative messages about your body may have started early in childhood. They might have come through abuse, or loneliness, or when you were told that some "baby fat" would define you. You might have had poor role models in the area of food and exercise. You also might have been influenced by cultural messages which gave you an unrealistic standard to strive for. Whether your dad called you fat, or your gym teacher made fun of you…Whether you invested hours into fashion magazines or online images which hooked you into believing that you simply were not good enough…It's time to face the root beliefs that have pulled you down.

Every person reading this has their own unique story. Your core beliefs about your health and body began with a message, or a person, or an experience. Negative beliefs grew over time into the normal state of your subconscious – one that affects everything you do.

My Story

I was a gymnast growing up and the pressure of having to weigh in and do body fat measurements at nine years old produced limiting beliefs about myself. I began to believe then that there was a direct correlation between how low my body fat was and my personal value. Then, when I hit puberty, I began to compare my healthy curves with girls who had a skinnier build, and I began to resent my muscular frame. Finally, an unhealthy dating relationship with a young man who put me down physically was all it took for me to downward spiral.

The fact is that even something very small can lead to big problems if we take hold of a lie and allow it to define us.

And as painful as it is, acknowledging the root of your thoughts is key to moving forward.

These negative thoughts are an enemy attack on your personhood, and oh how I want to see every person reading this to not only recognize them for what they are, but to begin to fight back!

We need to acknowledge and deal with this fact: there is no diet or exercise plan that can set us free if our core belief about ourselves is negative.

Does this resonate with you?

We will get back to these negative beliefs in Chapter Four, but first take time to do some honest journaling, and read a short chapter about why diets cannot solve our problems.

Journal it:

Because this is a very sensitive part of your journey, I suggest you take some extra time with journaling. I encourage you to be prayerful in this step, and take time to share it with a trusted friend if you can.

1. What have you believed about yourself and your body? Have you lived with some false beliefs that you just now realize have dragged you down? How does that make you feel?

2. When and where did these thoughts begin? Take some time to acknowledge this. You might want to journal a letter to someone from your past (just to keep for yourself) or even a letter to your past self. This is a part of your story…Though it is not the end!

monicaswanson.com

Diets Are Not The Answer
So Why Do We Keep Coming Back To Them?

If you understand how the cycles work, you should begin to see why diets can't solve our food and body image problems.

Most people reading this book have tried one diet plan or two (or 28!) only to be sorely disappointed later when you found out that it not only did not deliver on its promises, but it also left you feeling like it was all your fault. Perhaps it also left you in the end with more pounds than you started with.

But the funny thing is, people keep dieting. Why?

We live in a time where people are simultaneously obsessed with food, and body image. We also live in a culture of instant gratification. Dieting appeals to our conditioned quick-fix mentality. Even if it doesn't make logical sense (because it really doesn't) the diet industry thrives.

Boston Medical Center[1] reports that approximately 45 million Americans diet each year, and we spend $33 billion on weight-loss products in the pursuit of a leaner body. You'd think we'd all wise-up to the money-making machine that the diet industry is, but instead people keep trying…
Just. One. More. Diet.

But if you think logically, the concept of dieting really makes no sense. You simply cannot solve a problem rooted in a person's thinking and core beliefs by giving them a food plan to follow. It's like sticking a Band-Aid over a deep infection.

The diet industry has worked really hard to make us believe in diets, and when a diet doesn't work, to keep us coming back for more. But in the end, we are the ones who lose. (And I'm not talking about weight.)

Diets don't stop you from thinking about food. In fact, I would bet money that people on diets are thinking more about food than when they are not on a diet. Diet plans do not take a dieter's mind off of food.

The guarantees that diet plans offer rarely work out. If they do, then give it five years and tell me if it is still working out.

---

[1] http://www.bmc.org/nutritionweight/services/weightmanagement.htm

Note:

When a diet plan is successful in the long term, it is because the person who followed the diet developed new lifestyle habits which they embraced in their thinking. They committed to it for the long haul. At this point, I do not give the diet itself credit, but instead the person who was 100% ready for real change.

Journal it:

1. Have you turned to diets in hope of real life change? If so, how many? (You can be honest, this is just for you!) Did you experience positive results, and if so, how long did that last?

2. Has a diet ever freed up your mind from food or thoughts of your body? If so, for how long? Can you imagine a life free of dieting forever? What would that look like?

monicaswanson.com

Four Steps to Real Change
How To Get On The Thin Cycle

We have taken a good look at how our core beliefs lead to our thoughts which lead to our behaviors, which lead to our experiences. It's a cycle, and we're all on one, positive or negative. Like it or not.

Hopefully you've taken some time to consider where your negative beliefs came from, and the damage they have done. I hope that you are on the edge of your seat now, ready for real change.

We have already seen that dieting is not the answer…

But the good news is: you can get on the Thin Cycle! You can change the course of the rest of your life!

I did it, and I will show you how you can too.

As we saw, there are four steps in each cycle:

BELIEVE
THINK
BEHAVE
EXPERIENCE

Getting onto the Thin Cycle begins with your beliefs.

BELIEVE

Changing your false perceptions, or limiting beliefs about yourself is the key to the Thin Cycle. Replacing your old beliefs with an enabling truth will set the rest of the positive cycle in motion. *(An "enabling truth" is simply a new belief about yourself which is set in the positive direction you want to go.)*

The good news: *you* get to choose the beliefs that will shape who you want to be. We'll talk in a minute about what to do with your old beliefs, but for now let's focus on where you're headed.

Take some time to choose the honest and positive ways you would like to define yourself.

Begin by describing physically who you would like to be. Get practical and specific. If you could lose weight permanently, be fit, change some habits, and have a fresh start…what would that look like?

Whatever your personal pitfalls might be, imagine trading them in! If you obsess over your body or exercise, imagine being free from the obsession.

Cast a vision for the life that you would like to call your own. You might call these your new beliefs, or your enabling truths. *They are your new best friend.*

Visualize who you would like to be in six months to a year.

Take time on this step. It isn't as much about throwing out a number, like "I want to lose 20 pounds," but it is more about imagining the person you would be if you lost 20 pounds. It is about believing that this is the *"real" you* underneath the layers (literally and metaphorically.)

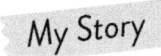

When I went through these steps, I began to get a vision for the person I wanted to be, and the lifestyle I wanted to live. I actually had admired other people, and used their lives as a model for what I dreamed of having…

Some things I imagined: being a lean, fit mom, playing outside with my children. Sitting down at the dinner table and eating the same meal as the rest of my family. Being out in public and completely focused on what was going on around me – not my body or food. Taking my children out for icecream and enjoying a treat right along with them. I imagined confidently carrying myself into future events, from upcoming holidays, to how I might look – and feel, at my children's weddings! I know that sounds far off, but it all really helped me to embrace this new way of living literally for the rest of my life.

Though it is fun to dream big and make grand plans for the new person we are becoming, I encourage you to be completely realistic in this step. Not only should you consider your God-given build, age, and any physical limitations you might have, but you should also consider your lifestyle. For example, family obligations or your work schedule.

If your goal is to be a competitive marathon runner or a swimsuit model, then your enabling beliefs will be very different from mine. And that's ok too. This is your life, so you get to choose your path and the corresponding lifestyle accordingly! The key here is to determine your values and your goals, and then prepare to think and live in alignment with those things.

If you have been at your ideal weight in the past, you might pull out a photo and hang it up. If you haven't, then turn to people you admire who have a similar build to you. Consider people who you would like to be more like in your relationship with food and your body.

Imagine yourself in 10 years. Or 20.

You are developing a vision for the person you believe you can become.

My Story

When I was going through this step, I actually committed to decreasing my workouts because I realized that working out five days a week as I had been doing was adding stress to my family life. I decided that three to four workouts a week was something that I could manage, and something I could likely do for the rest of my life! I had observed other women who were healthy and lean and only worked out only occasionally, so that built my confidence that I could do it as well. (I also considered how many women I knew who worked out religiously and still battled with their weight.) These were all important observations that I considered as I formed my new beliefs. They also helped me to be more objective as I moved forward in becoming who I am today.

I have a muscular build, so it wouldn't be wise to compare myself to a small-boned, super skinny friend. When I went through this process, I observed women who were around my height and build, who seem to have a healthy mindset with food, and a balanced lifestyle. I modeled after them.

In my personal observations and the interviews I have done, I found that people I most admire are not obsessed with food. Most of these women do exercise, but not compulsively. They couldn't tell you their exact weight today, but would claim that it hasn't really changed much in the past few years.

These women seem to enjoy all kinds of food, but if I'm watching them carefully, I would describe them as "careful eaters". They eat mostly small portions, and then enjoy a meal out, or a little indulgence on a special occasion. I never remember seeing these women stuffing themselves or binging. I see no evidence of them having a love affair with food.

So after observing these women, I decided: that's how I want to be.

And I dared to consider if I too, could be on the Thin Cycle. What if I believed and behaved like a thin person?

Then I committed to the enabling truths that would shape me.

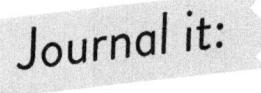

Journal it:

This is your time to envision the YOU that you hope to one day be.
Here is a list of helpful questions to ask yourself as you do this exercise:

What does the ideal you look like?
What would an ideal daily routine look like? (Be realistic.)
How much exercise/what kind of exercise would the ideal you do?
How does the ideal you eat when she is alone? Out with friends?
Is there anything that she does NOT eat?
How does she handle holidays, special occasions, etc.?
What does it look like when she overeats or splurges a little?

Once you have this person in your mind, call her by your name.

monicaswanson.com

THINK

Changing your false perceptions, or limiting beliefs about yourself is the key to the Thin Cycle. Your thought-life will naturally flow from your beliefs, but thankfully, it works both ways! Choosing how you think will build up and fuel the belief system that you are working on.

In fact, directing your thoughts is the greatest tool you have in this process, because your beliefs will be established by repetitive thoughts. So lean in close as this section will be the key to the changes you want to make.

From this day forward, you get to choose your thoughts.

In fact, you must regulate your thoughts to be successful in this process. Imagine putting all of the focus and energy you have previously put into dieting or exercise plans into the act of reprogramming your thoughts!

Begin to choose positive and affirming thoughts that align with the beliefs that you are developing about yourself.

When I first started this process, I imagined being the gate-keeper of my mind. I chose carefully what thoughts I would, and would not let in! I looked at that as my "job" for a few weeks.

We might as well face up front the fact that those old beliefs and thoughts will not go away without a fight. So, let's talk for a minute about how to handle the old thoughts when they show up.

OLD THOUGHTS:

As you are getting on to the Thin Cycle, you must begin to make a conscious effort to reject all of the negative thoughts that have brought you down:

Obsessive thoughts: Thoughts about what you just ate, or what you will eat, or how much you did or didn't workout, or how much your neighbor worked out. From this moment on, do not allow yourself to count a calorie, to overthink what you should eat next, or meditate on anything related to the stuff that has brought you down.

For many of us, these thoughts have become like an evil companion. They are comfortable because they have travelled with you for so long. For me, thoughts about food or exercise or my body were literally my waking thoughts and the last thoughts of my day. Counting my calories or comparing what I ate to what I should have eaten…Anticipating what I might eat the next day, or at an upcoming social event….It was all on my mind…All of the time.

Rejecting those thoughts was extremely challenging at first. I guess that is why I had tried every diet I could get my hands on before I finally was willing to face my true problem: I had a thought-problem.

The crazy thing is, we often feel some sort of control by holding on to our negative thoughts. Pondering our workout plans, or beating ourselves up for overeating make us feel like we are doing something productive, when in reality the thoughts just drag us down.

When I first started intentionally blocking all of my useless preoccupations, I felt anxious. I felt a bit like I imagine an addict feels when they go off of drugs. After all, my thoughts had been with me for years. I hardly knew what to think about without them! Kind of like the childhood bully that puts you down but you still let stick around until one day you grow up and realize what a total jerk they are.

> **Declare your mind and heart to be a no-bully zone.**

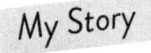

As I faced the overwhelming truth of the beliefs that pulled me down, I turned to God for the strength to face it. There were some deep-seated thought patterns that I realized would take spiritual power to overcome. You can find more about this part of my journey in the "Author's Note" at the end of this book.

NEW THOUGHTS:

We will replace all of the old, negative thoughts with new thoughts that align with our new belief system.

Your new thoughts should now be consistent with the beliefs that you have chosen to embrace. This takes time and effort.

You might write down positive statements about your health, your body, and your future. You can use inspirational quotes, or Scriptures. Each time a negative, or food-centered or body-centered thought enters your mind, speak to it: "You are GONE," and immediately replace it with something positive.

Some affirmations might come in the form of reminding yourself of how much better you'll feel when you are free of these obsessions. You might declare that you'll be so much more useful with a mind free to focus on other things. Speak the truth that you were created to be healthy and to live a full and happy life.

> In my 30-day "Thought Diet" companion guide (featured at the end of this book), I share three encouraging affirmations or quotes, plus one inspirational verse from the Bible for each day. I think you will find it to be super helpful through this part of the process. You can use these affirmations for breakfast, lunch, and dinner, or however you choose.

Since you have a list of specifics about the person you are becoming, it's not a bad idea to personally script out your thoughts.

For example, if one thing you want to define you is becoming consistent with exercise, and you feel tempted to skip a workout, try to objectively state, "This is who I am: I exercise four times a week, without question." If your goal is to trade in sugary desserts for healthier options after a meal, you simply say, "I'm going to choose fresh fruits over junk food. This is something I value, and I am worth it." Script out as much of who you want to be as you can! (Would you believe me if I told you this becomes really quite fun? It does!)

Because we're all coming from different places, this step will look different for everyone: Some of you might actually need to receive the freedom to eat dessert! You might need to give yourself permission to even enjoy food. You know yourself the best, so choose the words you most need to hear.

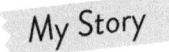

Even though my husband never judged me for anything I ate, I used to have such insecurities related to enjoying food that I accused him of judging me. Once I became free in this area, I have had so much fun enjoying food with my husband. There is a new thrill to ordering a juicy steak on a date and enjoying it without shame, even if he is the one eating something healthier! There was a time that I don't think I would have believed I could do that! And it all started with facing my beliefs head on.

This is the path to freedom, my friends:

Embrace your new beliefs. Think the thoughts.
Do it all enough and you'll find yourself changing on so many levels, before your very eyes.

> "As a man thinks in his heart, so he becomes."
> – Proverbs 23:7

Journal it:

1. List some of the thoughts that align with your new beliefs. What thoughts will help you move forward practically every day?
2. List some of the old thoughts that you are ready to go to battle against. One idea is to list them on a separate piece of paper, and then burn the list or tear it up to represent the end of them. This is a freeing step and you should take time to make it as official as you can!

monicaswanson.com

BEHAVE

Once you have chosen new beliefs about yourself, and know how to choose thoughts that are in alignment with your beliefs, the natural next step is to behave like the person you are becoming.

Your actions should reflect the person you are committed to becoming. Whatever you are personally working to change, it is now your responsibility to walk it out practically every day.

As you embrace new thoughts and beliefs, the corresponding actions will get easier and easier. However, keep in mind that your actions are also a valuable part of the cycle.

There will be times when it is your actions that will keep the cycle moving...Days where you struggle to believe what you have decided to believe, and where you are not "feeling all of the feelings". In those moments, simply choosing to walk out the behaviors will help you to keep moving in the right direction.

Pushing your plate away, or putting on your running shoes might just set you back on the cycle where you need to be. Choosing foods that you know align with the person you are becoming will become your new "normal".

The more objective, and unemotional about this process that you can be, the better. Remember, your eyes are on the horizon – as you imagine who you will be in six months to a year from now. Keep on the path and refuse to go back to old ways and thoughts.

> **Keep returning to the person you have envisioned becoming.**
> **Act like her. Eat like her. Think like her.**
>
> **And when you wake up tomorrow, do it again.**
> **And again.**
> **And again.**
> **Until one day you will realize that you ARE her.**

As you face each day, you will make decisions about food, exercise, and what your mind dwells on based on who you believe you are. You will need to practice the steps of rejecting negative thoughts and replacing them with positive, enabling truths until the negatives give up and quit coming back. One day they really will. I know. It happened to me, and I've seen it happen to others.

Please be kind to this person you are becoming! Give her grace. She is allowed to mess up occasionally, because she is human. Her greatest ambition is not perfection, but a new way to live.

Be strong! I can almost guarantee you that this process will not come naturally at first. The longer you have lived with unhealthy patterns, the harder this will be, so I plead with you to hang in there with it. If you slip up and think or eat like the person you used to be, you might find yourself studying where you went wrong, how to do better next time and on and on, and can I just say: STOP! Don't even go there! Your solution will not come through analyzing or obsessing about any of that, but it will come through literally moving on, rejecting the negative, and pressing on with positive affirmations.

Take courage!

PRACTICALLY SPEAKING....

Now, you are all set up with thinking positively, but here's the challenging part: We still need to eat, right? And exercise is pretty important for a long and healthy life. So we need to make decisions about these things. Like every day.

When I was going through this change from my own food/body obsession to freedom, I complained that unlike most addictions, when you struggle with eating or exercise issues, you cannot just "quit."

With that in mind, anticipate some challenges when facing food choices. You might be used to only eating what is on a diet plan, or maybe you have been in a bad habit of eating whatever is in front of you without thinking about it. If you're like I used to be, you might overthink everything you eat.

So...start simple! Do not get stressed out or anxious over whether you should start your day with toast, eggs, or oatmeal, just choose one! (toss a coin if you need to — the point is, don't overthink it!) If your goal is weight loss, of course you'll keep your portion small because that aligns with the new you.

Eat whatever you have chosen, put your plate away, then get on with life. Literally: get on with life! Get your mind off of the food as quickly as you can. You might need to be drastic at first: get out of the house – away from whatever is dragging you down. (The next chapter will cover some tricks and tips that you might find useful as you put this into action!)

If you value healthy eating (and I hope you do!) then I encourage you to choose healthy foods for most of your meals. If you are a guest at a home or eating out, remember you have the freedom to eat anything, just keep your enabling truths about yourself at the front of your mind.

My Story

I truly value healthy eating. When I am on my own I almost always choose whole foods, lighter options, and a lot of fruits and veggies. (As well as a bit of chocolate every day!) However, I value people and a balanced life even more than my healthy diet. For example, if I have a meal at someone else's home and they serve something that I would honestly not choose for myself, I eat it with gratitude. I may eat a small portion, but I will choose to enjoy every bite. There was a time where this situation would have stressed me out, or I would have made an excuse to only have salad, or to barely touch the food. But part of the "new beliefs" that I chose for myself was to be free in this area. I am so glad I made that choice!

Keeping my mind on the bigger picture has been a key to helping me in these situations. Really: one meal at a friend's house honestly won't change the scale when I weigh in six months from now, so why get uptight about it now?

So choose what you are going to eat, and as soon as you finish eating, discipline yourself to move on. Get busy with other things! Do your daily stuff, and even get absorbed in a hobby or activity that you love. This is the time to read awesome books, plan your next vacation, or become a volunteer. Learn photography, start a new Pinterest board, or take Great Aunt Martha our for tea. You name it –there's a whole to do with all of that free mental space!

As you do your things, continue to practice your beliefs and thoughts.
Over and over and over again.

I have friends who have applied these principles to their post-menopausal, changing bodies. They want to go into this next season with more muscle-tone, and more energy. By practicing the believe-think-behave-experience cycle, these friends are able to consistently practice the behaviors that will make them the strong and fit women they want to be in this next season.

I also have friends who have overcome eating disorders. Though they have been under the care of a medical professional (and if you have an eating disorder that is what you should do,) applying the believe-think-behave-experience cycle has helped them establish a new way to live, and a fresh vision for their future. They have found hope and freedom through realizing that they can actually carve out a new "normal" for the rest of their lives.

I could go on and on with examples of how this cycle can be applied to your life: from overcoming health issues, to an improved social life, to accomplishing health and fitness goals beyond your wildest dreams. Who says you can't do a triathlon? Who says it's too late to try yoga? I believe that applying a new mindset can change the entire course of your life. Starting now!

There is a real freedom to moving beyond the emotional side of thinking and eating, and making objective decisions about how you want to live your life. Begin to trust the process.

Next we will talk about the benefits of being on this new cycle…

Journal it:

1. Describe some new behaviors that define who you are becoming.
2. You might get specific with the types of foods you want to define you, the type of exercise you are ready to commit to, the type of lifestyle you want to live. What would an average day look like for you, given the season you are in and your new beliefs about yourself?

EXPERIENCE

As you are reprogramming your core beliefs, directing your thought life, and aligning your behaviors accordingly, the reward will be in your experiences.

It may not be immediate, but it won't be long before you see…feel…experience a different way of living! You will achieve physical goals. You will lose weight, or gain muscle, or be more fit. Be it weight loss, improved fitness, a healthier mindset, your goals are all within your grasp.

But just as valuable as all of that will be the satisfaction of walking with your head held high because you are becoming someone better: you will respect yourself.

You are on the path to a healthier, happier future. Your thoughts, actions, and beliefs will be aligned and consistent.

You will have plenty of opportunities to be challenged and grow. I encourage you to reframe your thinking to see slip-ups or challenging situations (travel, holidays, etc.) as a chance to prove that your mind is strong and your body will be ok!

My Story

A few years after I began living with new beliefs about myself, I stubbed my toe and broke a metatarsal bone pretty bad. This was right before holidays, and we were traveling to the mainland to see family. I had a moment of stress, thinking of all of the food I would be eating and wondering what would happen since I couldn't go running while we were on vacation like I normally would have done. I recognized my false beliefs then, and committed to taking a healthy mental approach to the trip.

As it turned out, I had the most wonderful holidays ever. I enjoyed all of the holiday food – though in moderation – and I also loved relaxing all month long, knowing that running wasn't even an option! My clothes never fit any different, so I'm guessing that I didn't gain any weight (I didn't get on the scale to check, because why would I?) I truly ended that month so proud of myself, and so empowered to continue to walk in freedom!

Believe in yourself as you make changes. This is not a quick fix, but a new lifestyle, and you will be so glad that you walked through it down the road!

Please remember: mistakes are part of this process and the truth is, even the people we look at as role models sometimes overeat, or make bad choices! But I also guarantee that you'll do this less and less over time. And one day it won't even be an issue at all!

My Story

I splurge on little treats pretty much every day, but I am no longer even tempted to over-eat or binge for emotional reasons. And because I do not count calories or analyze what I eat, there are days that I probably eat significantly more than other days – not because I am binging, but simply due to the circumstances of the day. The cool thing is that now I don't even notice it because I literally move on without a second thought. That means that one day of eating more never ever leads to another day (or a week, or month!) of overeating. It all balances out in time. And since I weigh myself about twice a year, I really wouldn't notice if the scale momentarily moves either direction. Now that is freedom!

Journal it:

Describe the experience you look forward to having six months to a year down the road. Dream of an upcoming holiday or vacation, and how it will look and feel to be experiencing it all with a different mindset and new habits of behavior. Revisit these imaginations often and use them as motivation for the changes you are currently making!

monicaswanson.com

Practical Tips and Tricks
Helpful Ways to Approach Major Challenges

CHALLENGE: WEIGHT LOSS

1. Embrace a new mindset!

If you're committing to these new mindsets, and your goal is weight loss, then learn to have some fun with the idea of swapping out a "diet mindset" for your new "freedom mindset". You see, when you diet, you are following a diet "plan" which tells you that you can eat a certain amount for each meal. A dieter's typical response to this is eating everything within those limits. *To the last morsel.* After all, the diet "promises" weight loss if you stay within those guidelines, so you might as well get in all you can. Right?

So, now that you are "free" to eat what you want, what if you try eating less? Most of us don't need a whole lot of food to stay alive and well, and since you're in the process of falling "out of love" with food, you can actually get by eating a lot less than you think you need. You'll probably feel really smart and sassy when you eat less than you would on a diet, just because you choose to! (After all, you're allowed to eat more later if you feel really hungry!)

Play around with things! Learn to go a little hungry now and then. You're going to be ok.

Practice these steps long enough and you'll join the ranks of those of us who often forget to eat because we're just busy doing life!

2. Find your own secret weapons.

Here are a few of my own: **Light breakfast!** Many people (myself included,) find that eating something light in the morning sets us up for a successful day. I know, I know—some people say that it is healthy to eat a big breakfast (and maybe it is,) but I do what works for me. Unless I'm out at a great restaurant (which I love to do, but rarely make time for,) I don't eat much for breakfast. I used to think I needed more in the morning, but after trying for a month or two to eat light in the morning, I found that my body adjusted to that and I did just fine.

Eating a small serving of oatmeal, or yogurt and fruit, or even a well-balanced energy bar is usually enough for me. Then I get busy and when my stomach is growling a couple hours later, I will enjoy another small meal or snack. This sets me up for a healthy-eating day.

The key is in your mind. Play around with things that help you feel and live positively.

Giving up night-time snacking: Because I was obsessed with food, I used to find myself drawn like a magnet to the fridge in the evenings. I just wanted one more snack before bed. Then another. And so on. I would tell myself: "I'm starting fresh tomorrow...I've already blown it today."

When I began working toward freedom, I just decided to make it a new habit to have a cup of herbal tea at night. I wouldn't even allow myself to consider eating after dinner. (After all, the woman I was becoming was not an obsessive night snacker, so why would I do that?)

It probably took me a full month to reject the temptation to snack and to just enjoy my tea, but over time that little habit became a very soothing night-time ritual. Now I rarely even think of food once the dishes are done, and if I do, I must be legitimately hungry, and I'll find something easy to eat. (It might happen once a month these days.)

Eliminate "Trigger foods": Some people need to begin this process by just cleaning out their cupboards. If eating one potato chip might throw you into a potato chip binge then get rid of the darned potato chips. No one needs them anyway. If you keep any food in your house that is a serious temptation or might trigger your old thoughts and habits, then as you begin this new season, I recommend you trash them. There will be a day (I promise!) where those same foods will not even tempt you any more. But until then, don't mess with them. If you can avoid restaurants or other places that drag you down, just be mature and make the right choice. Again, this is a process – be patient with yourself.

What about "Trigger Friends"? Now what to do with that friend that seems to always bring you down? You always splurge on sweets when you get together. Or she brings you a sweet treat on a hard day. Some of you might have friends that talk constantly about their weight or their latest diet, and you know this will bring you down. I recommend you let these people know that you are making changes that will make you a happier person. If they want to join you – great, if not ask for their support and respect. If you find that these friends just challenge you too much or pull you down, then this may be a season to take a break from those friends. You and your health and your mental freedom are worth it!

Journal it:

1. What are some of the practical danger zones that you know you will be facing as you change your thinking and body? Don't be in denial. Name them specifically.

2. What tips or tricks do you think you can apply to your areas of danger or temptation? Maybe something listed here, or maybe something personal to you. You are wise enough to come up with solutions to your problem areas! If it is hard to think of, imagine you have to give advice to a friend struggling with the same issue. Sometimes we are better at offering advice to others than we are giving ourselves advice! Whatever your concerns are, write down a way to target that area!

monicaswanson.com

CHALLENGE: EXERCISE ADDICTION

If you have been a slave to your workouts, you know what a burden it can be. I personally used to exercise at least five times a week, and feared that if I didn't, I would lose control. Part of being set free from all of my unhealthy mindsets included giving up my exercise obsession.

Your thought life will be the key to releasing your grip on workouts and accomplishing your personal goals.

> **If you live with a belief that loosening your grip on workouts will equal everything spinning out of control, then your actions will match that. One day off schedule, and you might overeat, feel bad about yourself, sit around, overeat some more...it's really a nasty cycle!**

But if you believe that your workouts are not the boss of you...then you can miss a few days, give yourself some positive self-talk, and cruise through it. You'll eat a little less knowing that you are burning a little less, and you'll learn to appreciate the extra time you just added to your life.

Some people fear that cutting back on workouts will lead you to quitting workouts altogether. *You're better than that! You can find balance.*

For those of you ready to step back from an unhealthy relationship to exercise, I want to encourage you to just do it. Be brave! You don't want to live the rest of your life burdened because of your relationship to working out. *(And for the love of your family/social life–trust me when I say that it's hard to be a friend or family member to someone who puts their workouts before people and other important things.)*

I'm not suggesting anyone should quit exercising. Exercise is healthy and should be a regular part of everyone's life, *for a lifetime*. But what we want to shed is the compulsive drive to exercise with an unhealthy mindset involved.

I shared a blog post with five guidelines to help you quit being a slave to your workouts. I think they are worth sharing here:

1. REMEMBER: It's widely acknowledged by pretty much every health and fitness expert that your **DIET** is the biggest factor in determining your body fat and weight. Most agree that your diet makes up about 80-90% of your weight maintenance goals. Just remember that and it will help.

2. As you decrease your workouts, you often actually lose weight. Sure, some of that is muscle, but often it is more than that. Truth: Less exercise will lead to less of an appetite. It might take a few days, but I find that when I am not working out, I can get by eating a whole lot less. In fact, so much less that I realize that the amount more that I eat when I am working out is probably more than the calories I burn on those days. Which (if I do the math) means that I am probably burning more fat on the days I don't exercise. Just an interesting thing to consider!

3. When you don't workout, you will have all the more energy to get things done. On the days I exercise hard, I find that I often want a nap later, and I am really tired at the end of the day. On days that I do not workout, I am powering through my days, often doing more cleaning and projects that require energy. So when it's all said and done, I probably burn as many calories throughout those days – PLUS I got stuff done. Double bonus!

4. Your workouts will rock! You will enjoy and go strong on your workout days all the more if you have a few days off in a week. After I've rested for two or three days, I am so amped to run hard, to workout strong. I love that! It is so much better than dragging myself through boring workouts every single day.

5. You will feel so proud. Trust me: something happens when you realize that you are not a slave to your workouts. You gain confidence in yourself. I know that is true for me – I feel so happy just knowing that I don't just look like I do (which isn't perfect, but is acceptable to me,) because I'm a slave to my workouts. I actually live a really fun, balanced life. *And I love being able to say that.*

Journal it:

If exercise addiction is one of your challenges, spend some time journaling in response to these questions:

1. In light of the facts shared in this book, do you really believe that you could take time away from your exercise routine, and NOT gain weight OR go crazy? How does this thought make you feel?

2. List a few ways that skipping workouts or taking more breaks would free you up to do other things or focus on other people/things.

3. What do you think is a realistic plan for your workouts in the future? You might include what kind of exercises you would like to do, or even how you would like your relationship with exercise to look. Maybe you would like to exercise more for enjoyment, and less out of duty. Maybe you would like to try some new things rather than feel obligated to do what you've always done because you feel like you have to.

The Resistance
Who This May NOT Work For, And Why

Change is hard. A radical change in your thinking and lifestyle can be really, really hard.

As much as I want freedom and success for every single person reading this, I also know that some people are not going to do anything with it. Some people will not be ready to move forward, and that is ok.

For me to be "ready" meant I had exhausted all of the other options. For me, "ready" meant I had walked through a lot of years all bound up in my thinking. It caused me anxiety, affected relationships, and certainly zapped a lot of joy from my daily life.

I don't believe it has to get to that point to make changes. In fact, the earlier you catch yourself with unhealthy mindsets, the easier it will be to take control back and change them.

Before I go on though, I want to address three reasons why you may not be able to make the changes I present in this book:

1. You don't believe it will work.

If you do not believe that this can work, it probably won't. The end. If I have not convinced you that your mind is the most powerful organ in your body, then you probably shouldn't even try this. You might still believe that the next diet will be your answer. You are absolutely welcome back if and when you come to the day that you are ready to take a step of faith and give real change a try.

2. It's too uncomfortable.

Some of you are convinced that I'm on to something, but the pain of letting go… of your exercise addiction, or your diet…or the control you feel over your body… is just too uncomfortable.

If this is you, then might I suggest you at least try taking some baby steps?

– Perhaps you can begin by becoming more aware of your thinking. This alone is huge. Notice what self-talk you are rehearsing each day. Maybe journal about it.
– If you are super into controlling your diet, you might switch up one part of your daily eating. Just small changes. See how it feels.
– If exercising is your drug of choice, you might try taking one extra day off a week. See if you survive. Experiment.
– Begin to be an observer of other people. Take an honest look at the lifestyle of those around you. Decide which ones look appealing and which ones do not. Make mental notes.

Taking baby steps might be just what you need to open up to real change. Perhaps dipping even your little toe in the water of change will help prepare you to dive in fully. And that's just fine. The change will be so much more beautiful when it's done in your own time!

3. Deep down, you are ok with yourself as you are.

I have a friend who diets constantly. She talks about her diets and jokes about her diets. Dieting has become a bit of her identity. I gave her the rough manuscript of this book, and after she read it we sat down and talked. We talked about her love for bread. We talked about how her weight fluctuates within about ten pounds. She told me how she jokes to her friends that if she were to lose twenty pounds, it would be dangerous because then she'd be "like a supermodel," and that would just be too much. It was funny. But she was a little bit serious. (And I had to agree—she's gorgeous.)

Then I stopped and thought about things. Finally, I said: "Do you think you might just be happy how you are? What if you decided that you like this weight and you like your bread, and what if you changed your thinking to determine that you will embrace and enjoy your current body – exactly how it is?"

And she said "That's kind of what I'm beginning to think."
I call that a breakthrough! I believe that she has found her personal "thin place."

> **Please hear this: If after reading this entire book, you look deep within yourself and decide that you just want to embrace YOU exactly how YOU ARE…and what you really need to change is habitual negative self-talk, then I will call that a success!**

Because here's the thing: it's still about the mind. If you've lived for many years talking negatively about yourself, and it has become a habit, then what I want most is to see you change that.

Ultimately, you want to have peace with yourself, and speak loving words that are consistent between your beliefs, thoughts, and behaviors. You will know if you are off track if any behavior (eating something, missing a workout, etc.) takes away your peace.

My Story

My current weight is a weight that my college self would have never accepted. I would have gone to extreme measures to lose five to ten pounds more before feeling ok. But today? My current weight, even with a couple pounds of fat (I'm not claiming to be heavy, but I do have some body fat I promise!) is totally acceptable. In fact, I have learned to associate the body fat I carry with the happy life that I live. When I see a little bump on my tummy, I am reminded that I am a mother. When I see a little jiggle on my thighs I remember how much fun I have on date nights with my husband, or having real ice cream with my kids.

Being fully alive and loving food (not being *in love* with food!) is something I am proud of.

Journal it:

1. Do you believe that the mindsets and actionable steps listed in this book could work for you? Be honest. Are you fed up with every other option and ready to try it? If the answer is no, journal that honestly. Include why or why not.

2. Are the thoughts presented here simply too uncomfortable for you to imagine giving it a shot? Perhaps these ideas have brought up memories or issues that are deep-seated and painful. Do you feel like you might need to talk to a counselor or therapist about some of this? Journal about any blocks or fears that you have when you consider changing your thought life in order to change your body and your future.

3. Perhaps you are beginning to realize that your biggest enemy is actually your thought-life itself, and you could be happy with your body as it is. If you are physically healthy, could it be that you might want to grow in gratitude of who you are and what you already have? If this is true for you, you might take time to journal a letter to yourself, offering grace and forgiveness for the years of rejecting yourself physically, or wasting energy striving to be something other than what you really know deep down is who you are supposed to be.

7 Special Occasions, Vacations and Real Life
Making It Real

> Here's one way to know if you are still "*in love* with" food, and how you're doing with exercise:
> How do you behave on vacation? On your birthday? A holiday?

HOLIDAYS

Food: Food is wonderful. I believe that food is a gift from God, and that there is nothing wrong with enjoying it. Especially if it comes in the form of a Thanksgiving feast with family, or a chocolate cake on your birthday.

However, a mind that is free from food obsession will not go crazy on Thanksgiving, or your birthday. *It just won't.*

Now that I am free, I will enjoy a piece of birthday cake or enjoy a special dessert on a holiday, but I have absolutely no desire to overindulge any more. *It's simply not a temptation.* It doesn't make me feel good.

Workouts: On Holidays I love to start the day with a workout. It just sets me up for a really positive day. If it doesn't fit our schedule, I am not thrown off or freaked out, but I do enjoy it when I can.

If holidays cause you to obsess over food, eat differently than you would any other day, or go extreme in either direction with your workouts, then you probably haven't really *broken up* with your unhealthy thought-life yet.

VACATION

When I am on a vacation, I eat about the same amount as I do any other day. I enjoy the feeling of taking care of myself. I'll look forward to trying new restaurants or indulging a bit in something special from a vacation destination – but only in moderation. (And I do that in my normal daily life as well.) *I don't see vacation as a time to blow it.*

I also really enjoy getting some exercise on vacation. I love to take a run through a new area, or find an exercise class to drop into. If it doesn't work with the family schedule, no big deal. But it is just who I am so I do it when I can.

> **If you use vacations as an excuse to blow it, or assume you'll gain back five pounds because you're traveling, that is a red flag that you're not yet free.**

This isn't about self control as much as it is about a very different relationship with food and exercise. It is about defining who you are, and remember: "who you are" goes with you wherever you go. Give yourself grace, but know that these things are an indication of your relationship with food and exercise. So be intentional every day. Including holidays and on vacation.

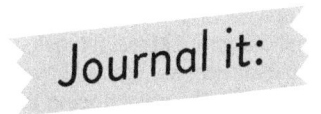

Journal it:

1. Up till now, how have you behaved in regards to your diet and exercise while on vacation? What has your mindset been? Do you see how this communicates a lot about your relationship with food and exercise?

2. Up till now, what has been your approach to holidays or special occasions? What does this say about your deep-seated feelings about your body and your relationship with food?

3. Can you imagine what it would look like to have a healthier relationship to food and exercise while on vacations or celebrating special occasions? Do you imagine you might feel empowered by making changes? What would this look like for you? (Describe it in as much detail as you like!)

Obesity, Special Diets & General Health

Does This All Still Apply?

I want to make a quick mention of special diets. I know that some people reading this have special diets due to a health issue like Diabetes, Celiac Disease and so on. Some of you have also chosen specific dietary restrictions due to your own moral or health convictions. You might be vegetarian or vegan. Regardless of your dietary restriction – no worries! You can still apply every principle in this book, while following your dietary guidelines.

If you are clinically obese, and are following a doctor-prescribed diet to help get your weight under control, by all means, do what the doctor says! I do believe that in time your goal should be total freedom from diets, but I also understand that in some situations, following a regimented plan will help get you to a healthier place. I still absolutely recommend following all of the steps outlined in this book along with a prescribed diet. The more you can get the mental side of things under control, the better you'll do with the diet plan you are following!

If you have chosen a dietary lifestyle and you are becoming aware that your motivation was more about control or a disguised attempt at weight loss, you might have some second thoughts at this point. Some of my friends have quit eating gluten, or meat, or any number of things in the past, hoping that would be the secret to weight loss, or that it would give them some sense of control. When they found true freedom, they decided not to restrict themselves completely from those foods anymore. They now enjoy freedom in their diet, though they are still "careful eaters". *(Their families appreciate how much easier they are to be around too.)*

My Story

I eat a little bit of everything, in moderation. I try to make the bulk of my diet healthy, "whole" foods, but I try to keep some variety in my life as well. I have decided that I will not eliminate any food group or type of food unless it is medically necessary. This approach keeps me healthy and free.

Five Days in My Life
Diet, Exercise and My Thinking

I have walked you through the steps that I took to retrain my mind and find freedom in my diet, exercise, and body image. I believe that by following them you too can find freedom, and begin to walk in a new lifestyle that will lead you to the ideal you.

I know it helps to have some practical examples of what all of this looks like in real life.

I already touched on how much of my mind was consumed with food, exercise and my body before I found a new way. Now I will walk you through a few typical days in my life, so that you can see not only what I eat and what kind of exercise I do on a typical day, but also the thoughts that go along with that.

Remember:

> **Being "free" in the area of diet, exercise, and body image, does not mean reckless abandon. There is a big difference between being "obsessed" and "careful."**

As for me and all of the women I interviewed for this book, there is an absolute "thoughtfulness," and "intentionality" in our relationship with food and exercise. However, the beautiful (might I say amazing and extraordinary and miraculous) thing is, as I walk in freedom in all of these things, the thoughts are 100% different than they were before. That's what I celebrate!

Here's a look at a few typical days in my life.

A WEDNESDAY IN APRIL

I wake up and go straight for coffee. A splash of half & half goes in it. I sit with my Bible and sip my coffee. Sometimes, I have a second cup. (Usually.) Once I have finished my coffee and used the bathroom (I'm giving the full story here) I make sure my boys are up and getting started on breakfast, devotions and chores, and I set out to run. I run for about 35 minutes, up some hills into the trails by my house. I return sweaty and gross. Then I shower.

I spend a little time with my preschooler, then drive him to preschool (about 4 minutes away,) at 9:00. By then my stomach is growling. I need to jump in to the homeschool day and I don't want to take time to prepare a breakfast, so I just grab a KIND bar. This is a quick, balanced, energy-filled snack which is usually enough to get me through until late morning. I eat it with a big glass of water, and get busy and forget about food.

By 11:00 I am hungry again. I blend up a smoothie of almond milk, one banana, 1/4 cup Juice Plus Complete (a balanced protein powder that has fruit and veggie powders in it) with ice. It's yummy and satisfying.

After picking up my preschooler at noon, I make my boys lunch. This is often heating up leftovers, or throwing together a quick PB&J. If the leftovers are yummy, I will often just make a small serving for myself as well, and eat it standing up in the kitchen while I serve them. (Yeah, you're supposed to sit. Maybe one day I'll actually do that!)

On this day though, I did not eat what they had but waited. My smoothie had filled me up. At 2:00 my stomach growls and I remember that I never really ate lunch, but I'm rushing out the door, so again, I don't have time to put something together. I eat a quick Greek yogurt and grab an apple to munch on in the car. (I'm headed to the kids' dentist and I know there is Starbucks next door. That's worth waiting for.) I take kids to their dentist appointment, and while they are there I sneak next door to Starbucks and get a grande soy latte. Extra foamy.

We are back home at 5:00 and Dave gets home from work but quickly grabs the boys to hit the beach for an evening surf. I marinade some chicken, put together a salad, and pull some crusty bread out of the freezer. I jump on the computer for an hour, and by 6:00 I am starving, but guys aren't back and dinner won't be served until at least 7:00. So, I pull two slices of jalapeno jack cheese from the fridge and grab about ten gluten free crackers. I make a nice little plate and bring it to my computer desk along with a Perrier water. I sip my sparkling water and enjoy cheese and crackers while I write or reply to emails. This seriously makes me happy.

When the guys are back, I put the chicken on the grill and toss together a big salad with black beans, chicken, corn, tomatoes, shredded cheddar cheese, and mixed greens. I toss it lightly with a ranch/bbq sauce mixture and warm the bread.

I eat a big salad, and a small piece of bread. I might have water, or some ginger tonic or even a small glass of red wine if Dave and I sit down together and I'm feeling fancy.

Sometimes I make dessert, but most often the kids are welcome to fruit, yogurt, or some other snack (because they are always hungry an hour after dinner.) Unless there is a dessert that I really love, I usually just have a small square of dark chocolate from my secret stash. And then sometimes one more. (Usually.)

Later in the evening I sometimes make a cup of tea or my hot ginger tonic. I rarely think about food before bed. I am tired.

THURSDAY

Thursdays are busier mornings for me because Levi goes to a different preschool and it begins earlier. No time to exercise. I do the coffee and half & half, and then focus on getting him fed and dressed and to school in Haleiwa by 8:30.

When I get home I make myself a bowl of hot cereal. About a cup of it, with about 15 almonds on top, a sprinkling of brown sugar (I love it), and some almond milk.

Homeschool, laundry, emails, Facebook… Time flies.

The boys are in and out of the kitchen (they help themselves to most food during the day,) and by noon I am really hungry. I am happy to remember that there is leftover barbecue chicken from the night before. So I toss a salad very similar to dinner the previous night. I drink a Perrier.

By 2:00 I am sleepy. I make a cup of coffee with cream and help myself to a miniature square of chocolate (or 2) from my stash.

After picking up Levi, we go straight to swim lessons and I drop other boys at the beach, and we all get home at 5. Boys have Youth Group and I just wasn't organized to make dinner (and I'm smart) because I know that Dave will take us to our local Mexican restaurant while two boys are in youth group.

At the restaurant, I eat a few chips and salsa. Not a lot. I drink a diet coke (I've cut way back on diet soda, but I do like it, and occasionally splurge.) I order a salad that is spinach, black beans, a tiny bit of cheese, and shredded chicken. It comes on a flat shell but I ask to have it without the shell. (I enjoy munching on a few chips before my dinner and don't need the shell in addition to that.)

After dinner the kids want gelato from the brand new shop next door to the Mexican restaurant. I'm really not hungry but man it looks good. I order Levi a small and know that he won't finish it. I take a couple small bites of his and that is completely enough. It is rich and delicious, but I know I don't need more. I order a decaf coffee and sip on that which I love after a meal.

FRIDAY

Friday's are like Wednesday's for me, so I usually count on exercising. But this day is different because my husband is dropping boys to surf and I need to go pick them up and my "me time" is not going to work. I tell myself that perhaps I can exercise over the weekend. (It does bug me a bit because I truly look forward to working out. But I let it go with a little self-talk.)

After coffee and running kids around, I make a smoothie with 1 cup almond milk, a banana, a handful of kale, and a small spoon of almond butter. It is filling and delicious.

I pick up Levi at noon, and then at home I ask my older son to make everyone PB&J's. I am off to run a couple quick errands and meet a friend for coffee. I know that the Coffee Gallery has one of my favorite salads, so I wait.

I meet my friend at 1:30, and I order a delicious quinoa salad with corn, garbanzo beans, and olives in it. We visit for an hour and before I leave I order a Chai tea with soy milk. I get home and have a super busy afternoon of running kids around. Fortunately I have some fresh fish in the fridge, so dinner is easy. I steam baby potatoes, grill fish, and make a big spinach salad with strawberries, slivered almonds, and some feta cheese. Dave and I drop boys at Youth Group, and come home and have dinner with a glass of wine and watch Shark Tank. We each have a piece of dark chocolate.

I love Fridays. :)

SATURDAY

Saturday morning is a surf contest. Hear me moan at 4:45 AM when the alarm goes off. I make coffee for the road, and Luke and I drive in the dark to the beach. By the time I get there my stomach is growling. It's only 6:30. I'm hungry but I have a long day ahead so I decide to eat an apple to ward of hunger a little longer.

By 8:00 I really am hungry, so I eat a Balance bar, and drink a bottle of water.

Surf contest days are often about a bunch of small meals. Snacking my day away is not my favorite, but it is hard to eat meals at surf contests. I packed Luke a PB&J, but I'm not the biggest fan, so just stay busy keeping him on his game, sun-screened, and communicating with Dave who is at the hospital.

I'm honestly a little hungry all day this Saturday. Starting the day so early often does that. But I'm not dying. I'm ok with it. I eat an orange around ten, and a handful of gluten free crackers that are salty and I love them. Then I eat a Larabar at noon. At this point I seriously wish I had packed something more substantial.

Finally, the contest is over at 2:00, and we take off. We stop for frozen yogurt on the way home, and I pile mine with fresh fruit and a couple sweet treats. I drink water all day long.

Finally home, around 4:00, I lay down for a power nap. (Driving home in the afternoon is the worst for me...)

I get up at 4:30 and jump in the shower. I make a cup of coffee, and jump on the computer for a few minutes.

Dave offers to bring home Thai food for dinner. (I do a little happy dance!)

At 5:30 he is home with green curry with fish, red curry with chicken, pad Thai with chicken, brown rice, and spring rolls. I eat a full plate without thinking twice. It is delicious.

Jonah had made brownies while at home all day, so I cut a small square of brownie for dessert.

I collapse into bed by 9:30.

SUNDAY

On Sunday I ask the family to go to the later church service with the goal of exercising on my mind. I take my time with coffee, devotions, and computer stuff, and then hop on the elliptical around 8:00. I put in 35 minutes, and I get a good sweat going. When I'm done I pour a small bowl of granola, mixed with plain cheerios, probably a cup and a half total. I top it with almond milk and raspberries.

After church, the boys beg to stop at our little local food truck: Shark's Cove Grill. It's hard for me to resist their vegan garden burger (on a poi bun, which is quite honestly more like Hawaiian sweet bread.) I eat the whole thing. I nibble on a few fries that the boys ordered and drink iced tea. It is all delicious.

I'm busy all afternoon responding to emails, finishing blog posts, catching up on laundry, and preparing dinner.

Friends come over at 5:00, and I put out some chips and salsa. I eat three or four chips. We all have dinner on the deck on 6:00. I made my white bean chicken chili, corn bread, and salad. I eat a small bowl of the chili, and top it with a bit of shredded cheddar cheese and sour cream. I have salad, but skip the corn bread.

Our friends brought a pie from Ted's Bakery (the best!) so I cut a piece in half to split with Levi. We all have coffee on the deck after dinner.

As you can see, no two days look alike for me. I handle each day, as it comes, and often each snack or meal as it comes. There are certain meals that I repeat three or four times a week (a bar for breakfast is probably the most typical way I start my day,) but there are no foods that I feel I need to ban from my diet. I am thoughtful about the foods I choose to eat, but I do not dwell very long on any food choice I make. That is only because I trained myself to be that way.

Author's Note
Thanks and Credits

It is my heart's desire that everyone reading this will be able to apply the practical steps I share, and find increased freedom and an improved relationship with food and your body. I have so much confidence that you can do it!

I know that each of our stories is unique, and though you may relate to some parts of my story, you have your own. And more importantly, we are all still writing our stories! The beautiful truth is that we are given the freedom to write the story of our choosing!

Before I wrap up this book, I want to give some credit to the sources of my inspiration…

Thank you God: As I mentioned in my story, I spent a lot of time in prayer as I went through my journey to freedom. For me personally, once I discovered how consumed my mind was with thoughts about food and my body, I became overwhelmed. I actually felt powerless to overcome the habitual patterns of thought that I was dealing with.

It was when I read Beth Moore's book, "Breaking Free" that I recognized the spiritual side to my battles. Though her book does not discuss weight issues specifically, it does talk about finding freedom from any mental issue that we might be bound up in. My food and body issues definitely qualified. As I applied the spiritual principles in "Breaking Free", I found it much easier to practically walk through the thought changes that I needed to make.

You may find yourself also feeling overwhelmed at this point, and if so I hope you turn to God wholeheartedly for change. (You may find Beth Moore's book helpful as well!)

One thing I am certain of: The One who created you knows you better than anyone, and I believe that He cares about all of the details of our life.

More thanks:

Judy Huf: My friend Judy has been a strong force behind this book. I'm pretty sure that she was the one who originally suggested I write the book, and she has held my hand through every stage of it! She has tested my theories, edited my grammar, and been there for middle of the night text messages when I was so excited to finally choose a title for the book (only to change it again by morning!) Thank you Judy for your hard work, sense of humor, and friendship. You are one of the most beautiful people I have ever known, inside and out.

Test Readers: To Shannon, Corinna, Paige, Catherine, Laura, Jules, Elaine, Kari, and my Mom… Thank you. These friends span the globe, and though I haven't met some of you in person, I adore you all! Your feedback was priceless, and your support has meant the world to me.

Josiah: Special thanks to my son Josiah for the cover photo and graphics. Josiah, your skills and creativity are only surpassed by your kindness and patience. Thank you for working so hard on a project that is the furthest thing from interesting to a teenage boy.

Gisele: Thank you for your detailed editing work, and your lovely formatting. You turned an ugly document with a lot of bad grammar into something much more pleasant to read. Bless you.
P.S. You inspire me in so many ways, and I am thankful God introduced us!

Blog readers: Thank you to all of my blog readers who have commented over time and encouraged me to finish this book. I know it isn't the "main thing" I write about on my blog, but through emails and messages I know that a whole bunch of you have been cheering for me along the way. Thank you! I love you all, and I do hope that this is the first "book" of many I will get the opportunity to write!

I pray for every person reading this, that you experience victory. Please let me know how you do, friends. I want to encourage you, and walk with you through your personal journey as you create your own story of overcoming, and finding a healthy, free life! You are welcome to email me your story of overcoming, or ask follow up questions related to your challenges. I will follow up with related posts on my blog, so I hope you'll subscribe there and make yourself at home! I do hope you'll email me your success stories at: aloha@monicaswanson.com.

With Aloha,

Monica

monicaswanson.com

… MONICA SWANSON

The 30-Day Thought Diet

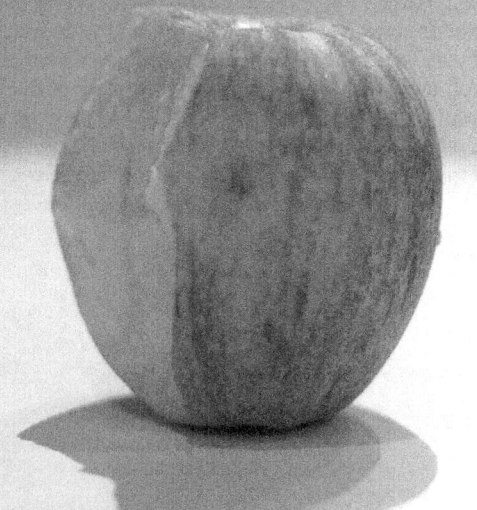

A companion guide to:

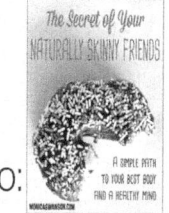

The Secret of Your Naturally Skinny Friends: A Simple Path To Your Best Body And A Healthy Mind

Introduction
What is the "Thought Diet"?

Aloha Friends!

This Companion Guide was written to help you along on your journey to choosing new thoughts which will help transform your beliefs, and in turn your body. These affirmations can be used for breakfast, lunch, and dinner, or however you find them most useful!

I wrote these affirmations because I understand that many people have habitually relied on diet or exercise plans to help achieve their weight and fitness goals. It is my hope that through the changes suggested in *The Secret of Your Naturally Skinny Friends,* people might find greater confidence to break free from diet plans which most often only cause us ton obsess further over our diet and body image. For anyone struggling to break free from following those plans, I thought this 30-day plan might be helpful. Each time you catch yourself meditating on what you should eat, or grasping for a sense of control, you might turn to these affirmations. If you can learn to focus more on regulating your thoughts than your food or exercise, you will be well on your way to a healthy mindset, and the body you are working toward.

Ultimately it is my hope that you will create your own affirmations that are personal and practical. I recommend you begin to write down positive thoughts, quotes, or verses that are supportive of the goals that you are working towards. As you go forward, also don't forget the powerful habit of rejecting any negative thoughts that might try to pull you down.

Your brain is the most powerful organ in your body! Do not underestimate the power of your thoughts, and don't take for granted the amazing gift God has given us in the freedom to choose them! Here's to a new way of thinking and living. Enjoy these 30 days, and when you finish them all, you can start from the beginning again! Please let me know how you're doing, or send me your personal affirmations at: aloha@monicaswanson.com

With Aloha,
Monica Swanson, author of *The Secret of Your Naturally Skinny Friends*

"As a man thinks in his heart so he becomes." – Proverbs 23:7

Day One

1. Who is this person I am becoming? (Take a minute to picture it!)
I will eat like that person.
I will make choices as if I had cameras on me and I was modeling just what that person that I am becoming eats like!
I can use my imagination today to create the future I want!

2. Each time my mind wanders to old habitual thoughts, I will be quick to reject them. Those thoughts are only going to tear me down, so I will battle them with all of my will.

3. "The best preparation for tomorrow is doing your best today."
—H Jackson Brown Jr, American author and inspirational writer

God's Word:
"Be strong and courageous.
Do not be afraid or terrified because of them,
for the LORD your God goes with you; he will
never leave you nor forsake you."
Deuteronomy 31:6

Day Two

1. Most experts agree that 90% of my results in achieving body composition goals has to do with how much I eat. Every meal that I practice healthy self control will pay off as I stay consistent.

2. Each day I need to go back to my personal Thin Cycle. What are the beliefs, thoughts, and behaviors that will lead to my goal experience. Commit to that cycle as a daily habit. It will pay off!

3. "If you have made mistakes, there is always another chance for you. You may have a fresh start any moment you choose, for this thing we call 'failure' is not the falling down, but the staying down."
– Mary Pickford, Canadian-born actress, co-founder of United Artists

God's Word:
"I praise you because I am fearfully
and wonderfully made;
your works are wonderful,
I know that full well."
Psalm 139:14

Day Three

1. Today is a new day, but added up with all of the other new days this is an exciting building block of the person I am truly becoming. This day matters!

2. I love the freedom to try new things and new approaches to my diet and life that might work for me. What one new thing might I try today? Is there a healthy food that I haven't tried? A new tea, or sipping on water with a yummy fruit or veggie in it? A new way to exercise as I go through my day? I get this one body and this one life so I want to live it well! I will practice gratitude today.

3. "Change your thoughts and you change your world."
– Norman Vincent Peale, author and minister

God's Word:
"May the God of hope fill you with all joy
and peace as you trust in him,
so that you may overflow with hope by
the power of the Holy Spirit."
Romans 15:13

Day Four

1. Speaking out loud about the person I am becoming will help me own it. Right now, I will name four things that describe the person I am becoming!

2. How will it feel to be at the next holiday event, summer barbecue or family wedding when I am free of the burdens that I have lived with? Take a minute to imagine what that day will be like: How I will look, feel, eat, and enjoy the day?

3. "Life is a succession of lessons which must be lived to be understood."
– Helen Keller, American author and activist

God's Word:
"You will keep in perfect peace
those whose minds are steadfast,
because they trust in you."
Isaiah 26:3

Day Five

1. An English Proverb says: "You may find the worst enemy or best friend in yourself." Be your best friend today!

2. Say it out loud: "I am beautiful. I am worthy. I have a future and a hope. I am worth taking care of. I don't need a diet book to tell me what to do. I can live freely and achieve goals because I have the confidence to walk out the life I want to live."

3. When I am tempted with a certain food, I can promise myself that if I still want it in a few days, I will come back and get it. Eating something that I don't feel good about on impulse is not wise, and I am learning to be wise. I don't want to be dragged down by those things any more. Now let's get the mind off of food and onto something beneficial!

God's Word:
"Trust in the Lord with all your heart
and lean not on your own understanding;
in all your ways submit to him,
and he will make your paths straight."
Proverbs 3: 5 - 6

Day Six

1. Keep this message from the book in your mind:
"There is no exercise plan or diet that will set us free if our core belief about ourselves is negative. The change must start with enabling truths, and positivethoughts. Focus on that and the rest will follow."

2. Each time I find myself dwelling on obsessive thoughts related to food, exercise or my body, I am reminded that this is actually a choice I get to make. Turning my thoughts away from unnecessary focus is a new habit that I excited to practice!

3. "I am not a product of my circumstances. I am a product of my decisions."
– Stephen Covey, author and motivational speaker

God's Word:
"Be on your guard;
stand firm in the faith;
be courageous; be strong."
1 Corinthians 16:13

Day Seven

1. Does the way I dress help me feel better about my body?
If I dress in a way that makes me feel good, I am all the more empowered to keep walking positively towards my goals!
Take the time to choose comfortable and flattering clothes and accessories. You are worth it!

2. No one can force thoughts into my head. I get to choose the thoughts and beliefs that I hold on to. If I have held onto thoughts for a long time, they may be habits now, so it is my job – my privilege, to deal with them. This is a task absolutely worth of my time!

3. "The pessimist sees difficulty in every opportunity. The optimist sees opportunity in every difficulty."
– Winston Churchill, Prime Minister of England during WWII

God's Word:
**"'For I know the plans I have for you,'
declares the LORD, 'plans to prosper you
and not to harm you, plans to give you
hope and a future.'"
Jeremiah 29:11**

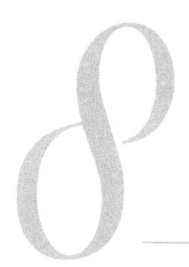

Day Eight

1. Who is that person I am becoming? Let's review a few qualities:
He/She is _____.
He/She enjoys _____.
He/She will look back later and remember herself as _____.
Add as many more statements as you need to affirm the person you are becoming!

2. Picture an open door. Behind it is a pile of the old thoughts, habits, and mindsets that used to drag you down. Now see yourself stepping through it to a new place. Imagine a lightness in you as you step through the door. Picture what is on the other side. Take a minute to describe what you see. Keep walking through that door today!

3. "When you get into a tight place and everything goes against you, till it seems as though you could not hang on a minute longer, never give up then, for that is just the place and time that the tide will turn."
– Harriet Beecher Stowe, American abolitionist and author

God's Word:
"The Lord is my shepherd,
I lack nothing."
Psalm 23:1

Day Nine

1. There is a big difference between *LOVING* food and being *IN LOVE* with food. Perspective is everything! A great goal is to be in a place where you can proudly *enjoy* food without it controlling you. If you are not there yet, believe that you will be one day. The hard work of regulating your thoughts now will get you there later!

2. No one can make me obsess over my body, and no one can stop me. I get to choose the focus of my thoughts. And the secret key is that when I obsess LESS, my body more quickly becomes what I really want it to be!

3. "It had long since come to my attention that people of accomplishment rarely sat back and let things happen to them. They went out and happened to things."
– Leonardo da Vinci, Italian artist, mathematician and engineer

God's Word:
"For now we see only a reflection as in a mirror; then we shall see face to face. Now I know in part; then I shall know fully, even as I am fully known."
1 Corinthians 13:12

Day Ten

1. It takes 30 days to form a new habit, and I am working on a lot of new habits right now. I need to be patient with myself, and trust that I can unlearn some thoughts and behaviors, and learn some new ones!

2. There are so many things that I have always assumed to be true that simply are not: That my weight must always be a struggle. That a happy and free life is for "other people." I cannot wait to live the rest of my life believing truths, not lies. This is just the beginning!

3. "When everything seems to be going against you, remember that the airplane takes off against the wind, not with it."
– Henry Ford, American industrialist and founder of Ford Motor Company

God's Word:
"Consider it pure joy, my brothers, whenever you face trials of many kinds, because you know that the testing of your faith develops perseverance. Perseverance must finish its work so that you may be mature and complete, not lacking anything."
James 1:2-4

Day Eleven

1. If I can unlearn a few bad habits each week, over the next year I will have an entirely new set of habits – good ones! I am excited to be discovering new ways to approach things! From food to exercise to how I relate to others – I get to decide what my life will look like. This is a privilege!

2. Keep returning to the person you have envisioned becoming.
Act like her.
Eat like her.
Think like her.
And when you wake up tomorrow, do it again. And again. And again.
Until one day you will realize that you ARE her.

3. "The great thing in this world is not so much where you stand, as in what direction you are moving."
– Oliver Wendell Holmes Sr, American physician, poet and professor

---

God's Word:
"Because of the Lord's great love we are not consumed,
for his compassions never fail.
They are new every morning;
great is your faithfulness."
Lamentations 3:22-23

Day Twelve

1. Just a few small bites with a big glass of water will sometimes satisfy you enough to make it to the next meal. Experiment with a little hunger. Be comfortable with some tummy rumbles. Get to know your body!

2. Sometimes doing light exercises throughout the day helps keep your mind focused on a healthy lifestyle. While you clean up the kitchen or do other light housework, you can do leg exercises, kegels, abdominal squeezes, etc. Working on the positive helps us not focus on the negative!

3. "The best day of your life is the one on which you decide your life is your own. No apologies or excuses. No one to lean on, rely on, or blame. The gift is yours – it is an amazing journey – and you alone are responsible for the quality of it. This is the day your life really begins."
– Bob Moawad, author and motivational speaker

God's Word:
"What, then, shall we say in response to these things? If God is for us, who can be against us?"
Romans 8:31

Day Thirteen

1. There will be a day where I'll wake up so excited and invested in my day that I don't even stop to think about food, exercise, or my body. In fact, I'll hardly remember what it was like to be obsessed with the old things. I must trust that those days are coming!

2. Please remember: Mistakes are part of this process and the truth is that even the people we look at as role models occasionally overt, or make bad choices. But I also guarantee that you'll do this less and les over time. And one day it won't even be an issue at all!

3. "It's not whether you get knocked down. It's whether you get up again."
– Vince Lombardi, American Football Coach

God's Word:
"Taste and see that the LORD is good;
blessed is the man who takes refuge in him."
Psalm 34:8

Day Fourteen

1. I get to decide who I am, including what I do and do not put in my body. What has dragged me down before? I will name it and decide that until my mind is truly free, I will remove that from my options. I am worth making some drastic decisions for!

2. Most people who seem to be "naturally skinny" have days where they eat more than others, but it all evens out over time. They don't dwell on it when they overeat. They move on, and most of the time they eat a light diet.

3. "Live each day as if your life had just begun."
– Johann Wolfgang Von Goethe, German writer and statesman

God's Word:
"Therefore, since we are surrounded by such a great cloud of witnesses, let us throw off everything that hinders and the sin that so easily entangles, and let us run with perseverance the race marked out for us."
Hebrews 12:1

Day Fifteen

1. Stand tall! Check your countenance and your posture. Keep speaking positive thoughts to yourself because you *ARE* headed somewhere and you will be so proud down the road. Sometimes it takes faking our confidence a bit before we really believe it. So, stand tall!

2. In six months, what my body looks like and how I feel will be a result of all of my days put together. Dwelling too much on one meal or even one day is not the answer. Just keep living and the results will come in time. I need to make new habits and keep my eyes on the horizon!

3. "Many of life's failures are experienced by people who did not realize how close they were to success when they gave up."
– Thomas Edison, American inventor and businessman

God's Word:
"No temptation has overtaken you that is not common to man. God is faithful, and he will not let you be tempted beyond your ability, but with the temptation he will also provide the way of escape, that you may be able to endure it."
1 Corinthians 10:13

Day Sixteen

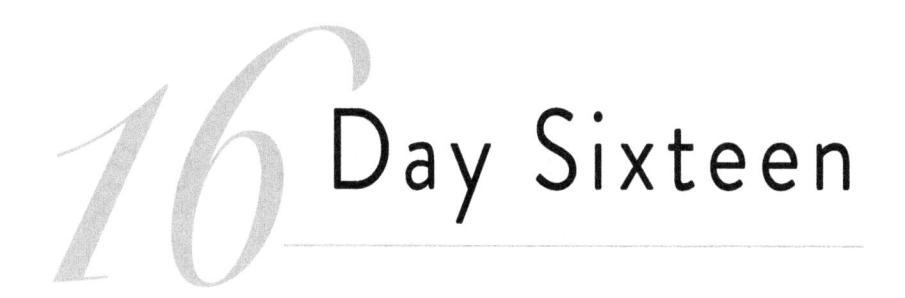

1. There is a saying: "Nothing tastes as good as being thin feels." This may be true, but even better would be to say: "Nothing tastes as good as it feels to be healthy and free from mental obsessions."
Be empowered today! Think before you eat, and be intentional.

2. Part of loving myself is feeding myself the things that my body asks for, and that I will enjoy. Too much of anything will not be good. I get the honor of making good choices!

3. "Courage doesn't always roar. Sometimes courage is the little voice at the end of the day that says I'll try again tomorrow."
– Mary Anne Radmacher, writer and artist

God's Word:
"So do not fear, for I am with you;
do not be dismayed, for I am your God.
I will strengthen you and help you;
I will uphold you with my righteous right hand."
Isaiah 41:10

Day Seventeen

1. Have I discovered some "trigger foods" that I need to eliminate from my life? Is anything in particular drag me down? Maybe I have some "trigger friends" that I need to talk to or take time away from. What practical steps can I take to more effectively achieve my goals?

2. I will continue to focus my eyes on the future – not tomorrow, or the next day, but six to 12 months from now. I am certain that my consistency – over time, will pay off. The person I am becoming will be so beautiful and free!

3. "If you hear a voice within you say 'You cannot paint' then by all means paint, and that voice will be silenced."
– Vincent Van Gogh, Dutch painter

**God's Word:
"I will instruct you and teach you
in the way you should go;
I will counsel you with my loving eye on you."
Psalm 32:8**

Day Eighteen

1. I am worth this! My future is worth this! The person I will be one day will be so glad that I dedicated time and effort to changing unhealthy mindsets and developing new ones. I will not feel guilty for taking care of myself.

2. Name three things you have done well this week in the area of your thinking, your eating, and your relationship to your body. Focus on the progress, not any mistakes! Keep going – this is a new way to think and live!

3. "Go confidently in the direction of your dreams. Live the life you have imagined."
– Henry David Thoreau, American author and philosopher

God's Word:
"Peace I leave with you; my peace I give you.
I do not give to you as the world gives.
Do not let your hearts be troubled and do
not be afraid."
John 14:27

Day Nineteen

1. Knowing my weaknesses is a big part of the battle! If I am aware of a challenging scenario, I can be better equipped to be ready to manage them well. This battle will not last forever but it is worth fighting until it new ways become new habits!

2. Grace is the one thing we all need every day. Even if it takes me a a year to figure out this new way to live, I will do it. With grace. Giving up is not an option. I will move forward full of confidence that I am headed to a new place and I am excitedto get there!

3. "There are those who look at things the way they are, and ask WHY…I dream of things that never were, and ask WHY NOT?"
– Robert F Kennedy, American politician and senator

God's Word:
"For the Spirit God gave us does not make us timid,
but gives us power, love and self-discipline."
2 Timothy 1:7

Day Twenty

1. Here's one way to know if you are still *in love* with food, and how you're doing with exercise: How do you behave on vacation, holidays, or special occasions? Keep yourself in check. Be honest. Seek change where you need it!

2. Wherever I am in my journey, I know that I am moving towards a happier, healthier future. Whether I have ever believed that I can live free of diets and obsessions or not, the truth is: I CAN. If I need to repeat that to myself a million times I will. It is truth, and I am on my way to living it out.

3. "My mission in life is not merely to survive, but to thrive; and to do so with some passion, some compassion, some humor, and some style."
– Maya Angelou, American author and poet

God's Word:
"Cast your cares on the Lord
and he will sustain you;
he will never let
the righteous be shaken."
Psalm 55:22

Day Twenty-One

1. I want to behave in private the same way I would if I were in front of others. That is taking care of myself, taking pride in myself. In the same way, I should be comfortable and confident publicly enjoying food and my body. It works both ways when I am a consistent person living a life I am proud of.

2. Sometimes just asking "Am I really hungry?" will help determine if I really need to eat, and how much. Drinking a glass of water or sipping on tea might be all I need! Learning to listen to my body is a huge key to making peace and enjoying a naturally thin future.

3. "It is in your moments of decision that your destiny is shaped."
– Tony Robbins, Motivational speaker

**God's Word:
"Whatever you do, work at it with all your heart,
as working for the Lord, not for human masters."
Colossians 3:23**

Day Twenty-Two

1. Remember: Being "free" in the area of diet, exercise, and body image, does not mean reckless abandon. There is a big difference between being "careful" and being "obsessed."

2. I'm so worth taking the time for! Do I need some fresh air? Some exercise? A healthy meal? Setting aside time and energy to fill my own tank will only help me serve the people in my life! Some of us need to find NEW and healthy ways to fill our tanks. Do it!

3. "Everyone has inside of him a piece of good news. The good news is that you don't know how great you can be! How much you can love! What you can accomplish! And what your potential is!"
—Anne Frank, diarist and writer during WWII

**God's Word:
"Cast all your anxiety on him because he cares for you."
1 Peter 5:7**

Day Twenty-Three

1. Delayed gratification is a character quality that spills over into all areas of life. It can serve us so well if we practice it and make it a lifestyle habit. Where might I practice delayed gratification today?

2. When thoughts creep in that try to discourage me or make me doubt that I am on the right path, I will literally force them out of my mind and replace them with positive thoughts. Who needs prayer now? Who can I jot a note to? Changing the channel in my mind is simply self control in my thinking. I can do this!

3. "You change your life by changing your heart."
– Max Lucado, Christian author and speaker

God's Word:
"'If you can'?" said Jesus. "Everything is possible for one who believes."
Mark 9:23

Day Twenty-Four

1. If you could step outside of yourself and see yourself from a friend's eyes, what might you say to encourage yourself? What do you most need to hear now? Speak it out loud. Learning to encourage yourself is a great life skill!

2. Passing up opportunities to eat things that I don't really want or need is so empowering. Saying, "No, thank you," to a snack or treat means I am saying yes to something I have purposefully chosen later!

3. "It always seems impossible until it's done."
– Nelson Mandela, African statesman and polical revolutionary

**God's Word:
"So encourage each other and build each other up, just as you are already doing."
1 Thessalonians 5:11**

Day Twenty-Five

1. Have I discovered any mindsets or thought patterns recently that I hadn't even realized I had at first? It is never too late to address false thinking and determine to change thoughts that creep in. Go back to the Thin Cycle each time you need a reminder! We are human, and this is a continual process when you are trying to live your best life!

2. Have you begun to identify with the Thin Cycle yet? Remember that your mind is your most powerful weapon. YOU get to choose which cycle you are on, and your body will follow. Enjoy the ride!

3. "Though no one can go back and make a brand new start, anyone can start from now and make a brand new ending."
—Carl Bard, Scottish theologian

God's Word:
"And we know that all things work together for good to those who love God, to those who are the called according to His purpose."
Romans 8:28

Day Twenty-Four

1. My body is a gift and taking care of it is a privilege. I should feed it thoughtfully, appreciate it, and enjoy it every single day!

2. Ever wonder why there are so many diet books out there? A new one pops up every day! It is because no diet has ever proven to be truly successful. 95% of people who lose weight dieting, will gain it back within the year. The only diet that will ever work for the long term is lifestyle changes. And you can only sustain lifestyle changes with a healthy mind!

3. "Challenges are what make life interesting and overcoming them is what makes life meaningful."
– Joshua J. Marine

God's Word:
"For our light and momentary troubles
are achieving for us an eternal glory
that far outweighs them all."
2 Corinthians 4:17

Day Twenty-Five

1. Always remember, if you begin to struggle with old habits, you can return to the Thin Cycle and focus on your enabling beliefs and new thoughts. It may take doing this over and over before habits are really engrained. Take this process as seriously as you would any other life change process. The freedom you are headed into is very real and will bless you and so many others!

2. Remember: "Naturally skinny" people are not thinking about food all of the time. They are not obsessing over what they just ate, what they are about to eat, or what YOU are eating. They really don't care."

3. "The most courageous act is still to think for yourself. Aloud."
– Coco Chanel, French fashion designer

God's Word:
"Being confident of this, that he who began
a good work in you will carry it on to completion
until the day of Christ Jesus."
Philippians 1:6

Day Twenty-Eight

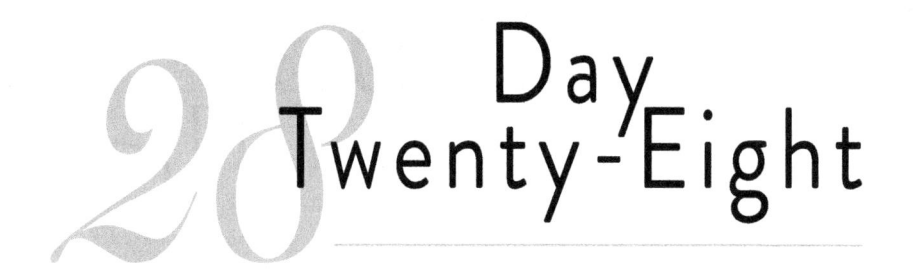

1. Name some positive changes you have seen in yourself since you began to change your thinking and your habits. List them out loud, or on paper—but make sure to take note of them! Give yourself credit, and appreciate your progress!

2. What are a some of the things I look forward to in six months to a year? Is there a physical goal that I have? (Name it!) Is there someone I can't wait to be with because of how different I am living now from before?

3. "Freedom is not the absence of commitments, but the ability to choose – and commit myself to – what is best for me."
—Paulo Coelho, Brazilian novelist

**God's Word:
"Rejoice in the Lord always.
Again I say, rejoice!"
Philippians 4:4**

Day Twenty-Nine

1. Think on this quote from the book: "I wondered: Why had I spent half of my life obsessing over diets, exercising compulsively, and completely preoccupied with my body, if I actually could achieve my goal weight by letting go of all of that?"

2. Name one positive experience you've had with food over the past month? Have you allowed yourself to have something that you used to consider "off limits" and enjoyed it? Have you said "no" to something that used to be hard to resist? Notice some of the progress you are making! Give yourself credit and lots of love.

3. "If I had to select one quality, one personal characteristic that I regard as being most highly correlated with success, whatever the field, I would pick the trait of persistence. Determination. The will to endure to the end, to get knocked down 70 times and get up off the floor saying, 'Here comes number 71!'"
– Richard De Vos, American businessman

God's Word:
"Let us then approach God's throne of grace with confidence, so that we may receive mercy and find grace to help us in our time of need."
Hebrews 4:16

Day Thirty

1. What have you learned about yourself through the first month of changing your thoughts and habits? Is there an area you realize you especially need to tackle as you keep going? Have you figured out some weak points, or areas of challenge? Great! That is how to keep improving. You're on your way – don't give up!

2. Speaking positively *TO* yourself is such a great tool. Speak it quietly and out loud! Tell your family that you are proud of yourself for taking the right steps. Declare your war on negative thoughts. Speak truths that will build up your confidence and inspire others to do the same!

3. "You gain strength, courage and confidence by every experience in which you really stop to look fear in the face. You are able to say to yourself, 'I have lived through this horror. I can take the next thing that comes along.' You must do the thing you think you cannot do."
– Eleanor Roosevelt, American politician, diplomat and activist

God's Word:
"Peace I leave with you; my peace I give you. I do not give to you as the world gives. Do not let your hearts be troubled and do not be afraid."
John 14:27

Made in the USA
Middletown, DE
20 October 2020